A history of disability in England

A history of
disability in England

from the medieval period to the present day

Simon Jarrett

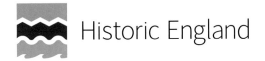
Historic England

Published by Liverpool University Press on behalf of Historic England, The Engine House, Fire Fly Avenue, Swindon SN2 2EH
www.HistoricEngland.org.uk

Historic England is a Government service championing England's heritage and giving expert, constructive advice.

The views contained in this book are those of the author alone and not Historic England or Liverpool University Press.

First published 2023

ISBN: 978-1-80207-855-8 hardback

British Library Cataloguing in Publication data
A CIP catalogue record for this book is available from the British Library.

Typeset in Charter 9/11

Page layout by Carnegie Book Production

Printed in the Czech Republic via Akcent Media Limited

Front cover: Matthias Buchinger, a phocomelic man.
[Etching by G. Scott, 1804. Wellcome Collection. Public Domain Mark]

Contents

Dedication: For Joan Jarrett, 1921–2021.
Also for Dianne, and of course for Hana.

The history of disability

This book offers a general introduction to the history of disability, predominantly in England, from the medieval period through to the present day. It provides a general overview of the subject, as well as a starting point for anyone who wishes to explore the field further and who may wish to extend their knowledge in particular areas of interest to them.

Before embarking on such a history, we must first answer the question, why a history of disability?

To understand and increase our knowledge about disability in history is important for several reasons. As the book will demonstrate, disabled people have always been a part of society and have had widely differing life experiences. These have varied both over time and between different individuals, places and groups. Such life experiences tell us much about attitudes within particular societies – most particularly the status of people who are seen as deviating from some sort of norm, either bodily or mentally. From this we can gain insights into concepts of belonging, community, humanness and morality in particular societies at particular times.

Sometimes the history of disability is described as a hidden history. This book will argue that it is no such thing. The history of disabled people is often in front of our eyes, yet we frequently choose to ignore it, or simply do not see it. Accounts of daily life, events, art, literature, family histories and political debate have always featured disabled people who are there for all to see, but too often observers, particularly non-disabled observers, gaze straight past them.

This experience is not unique to disabled people. Many other groups, although undeniably present, have been ignored or erased from historical accounts at times because they are seen as people who do not matter. These groups have included the poor, women, black and other 'non-white' groups, and LGBTQ+ people. Much excellent work has been done in recent decades to rescue and tell the histories of these groups, and it is gratifying that at last the history of disabled people is now also being told by a growing number of talented historians, some of the best of them historians who are disabled themselves. Such stories need to be told because if history is not about everyone then it is not about anyone. To deny certain groups of people a history is to deny them their humanity, and is a failure to recognise the interconnectedness of all those who form the complex networks of human societies. Such groups need to be rescued, to use the words of the famous historian of working-class culture E P Thompson, from the enormous condescension of posterity.

Finally, whatever wider arguments we may make for the importance of the history of disability, we should remember that this is at heart an interesting story. It is the story of numerous individuals who have often had to pit themselves against huge obstacles placed in their way because of the type of person they were born as, the type of person they became through accident, illness or circumstances, or the type of person they were perceived as. How they have done this, how they have seen themselves, how they have been perceived by others, how society has treated them, how they have influenced society – all of this is an endlessly fascinating one-thousand-year narrative.

In a short book, which seeks to tell the story of many different people with different forms of disability over a millennium, it is inevitable that far more must be left out than has been left in. It is unavoidably a potted history, and there have been many difficult decisions about which life stories, events and issues to include and which to exclude. The book could have been many times longer and still not included everything that deserves to be part of it. I can only reiterate that this account should be seen as a starting point, a gateway into a fascinating realm of history.

***

What do we mean by 'disability'? And, what do we not mean? Unpromisingly, there is no universal agreement on what constitutes a disability. It is important to note that it is only since the 20th century that there has been the general category of 'disabled' that is in use today to encompass a very wide range of physical and mental impairments. Such a wide category would not have been recognised or understood prior to the mid-20th century when groupings, if they were used at all, derived from particular types of disability, such as blindness, deafness, mental impairment or physical impairment.

One disability organisation active in the British cultural sector, Accentuate, describes the range of conditions that are grouped under the label of disability as 'wheelchair users, people with mobility problems, hearing impairments, vision impairments, deaf people who use British Sign Language (BSL), people with learning disabilities, those experiencing mental ill health, neurodiversity, other non-visible impairments and chronic health conditions'. They also talk about 'deaf and disabled people', hinting that deafness is a category that not all deaf people see as a disability.

There is always debate about what, or who, is grouped under the disability umbrella. For example, are chronic health conditions such as diabetes disabilities or illnesses? Is neurodiversity, which is used as a general category that includes autism, a disability, or are such conditions better described as a certain type of mind? What constitutes a non-visible impairment, and is it always a disability? Should mental conditions, such as mental ill health and learning disability, be grouped together with physical disabilities, or indeed with each other, given that they represent such radically different life experiences? There are many other similar debates.

Historically, a condition might be categorised as a disability in one age but not in another, as is discussed in detail following this introduction. Leprosy was so prevalent in the medieval period, and had such disabling consequences for people, that it can fairly be seen as a disability category at that time, but being far less prevalent and more treatable today, it can no longer fall meaningfully into the disability category. Autism has only been given diagnostic status as a disability in the period since the 1940s. While we may think we can recognise the characteristics of autism in individuals from before this period, it is very hard, and foolish, for us to try to diagnose them as such from our contemporary perspective. Further, to do so has little meaning for people who lived in a period when such a condition was not even conceived of, and its characteristics were not seen as a disability. Such 'retrospective diagnosis' risks imposing our modern propensity to diagnose and categorise on earlier periods. These changing definitions and understandings are discussed below in the discussion section, 'The shifting borderlands of disability' (p 8).

However, despite these potential pitfalls, to write this book it has been necessary to make some decisions about what to include as a disability and what not to include. The book covers therefore all types of physical impairment, as well as mental illness and learning disability. It also includes blindness and deafness, both from birth or acquired, and severe visual and hearing impairments. It considers leprosy as a disability in the medieval period because of its significant and widespread disabling consequences, but not in later periods when these consequences were generally far less severe. Otherwise, diseases such as smallpox, typhoid, diabetes or syphilis, for example, are not considered as disabilities, although of course they have always had disabling consequences for some.

These choices are not intended to assert a definitive statement on what constitutes a disability and what does not. It is not within this author's capacity or gift to make such pronouncements. Important debates and discussions on the definition of disability take place continuously among activists, theorists, historians and policy makers, and the book attempts in places to describe some of these debates. It is ultimately for the interested reader to investigate and hopefully participate in these discussions, and to form their own opinions. Nevertheless, the book must set some definitional boundaries and be clear about what categories are implied by the word disability that appears in its title, so these are the decisions that have been made. In a relatively short general overview over a long time period the choices make no claim to be either comprehensive or definitive.

Most controversial perhaps is the decision to include mental illness and learning disability under the general disability category. However, in telling the history of this subject it is almost impossible to tell the story of physical disability without including the story of what has been designated as mental disability or mental illness – the two have been brought together in legislation, asylums, other institutions, health and social policy, and public opinion in various ways over the centuries. It is at times almost impossible to separate them in the historical narrative. It is in this way that we see a wider cultural meaning of disability which implies that those designated as disabled are those who do not fit into prevailing bodily or mental norms, and are therefore bestowed with an outsider status that marks them out as not fully belonging.

Language

Any history of disability must grapple with the serious question of language. Much terminology that has been used to describe disability in the past has become offensive and hurtful language today. The litany of past disability language tells its own story: 'leper', 'cripple', 'spastic', 'defective', 'idiot', 'lunatic', 'moron', 'cretin', and so it goes on. The list seems endless. It is telling that so many of these words have become words of insult, revealing something of the marginalising and hostile social atmosphere which disabled people have so often had to endure. Most language begins as a socially neutral or clinical term, but quickly passes into the street language of insult or humiliation.

This poses a dilemma to any historian, of whether to use such language when it carries such negative and hurtful connotations. Not using such terms, and replacing them with modern terminology, creates two problems. First, it is ahistorical. To write about learning disabilities in the medieval period has little meaning – at the time there was no concept of learning disability as we understand it today. Most people were non-literate and 'intelligence' was not the defining characteristic for belonging that it has become today. There was, however, a concept of an 'idiot' at this time, a word which did not carry the weight of insult it does today, and which denoted a person with some limitations of mental faculty, who nevertheless invariably lived, worked and was supported within the community into which they were born. Similarly, the medieval word 'creple' did not carry the pejorative and hurtful tones which, as cripple, it does today, but was a relatively neutral term to describe someone with impairment of the limbs. Cripple was used as a self-descriptor by people with physical impairments well into the 20th century, and the campaigning *National Cripples Journal* did not change its name until the 1960s. It is also important not to assume that modern terminology has bucked this process and that the language we use today will always be acceptable. Language changes in uncontrollable and unpredictable ways, and the language deemed acceptable today has a high, indeed almost a certain, chance of being seen as unacceptable, insulting or inappropriate in the not-too-distant future. This is because just as disability is a shifting concept, so is the language that describes it, along with the social factors that determine how language is used and the meanings it conveys.

For these reasons this book uses historically accurate language. Where a word has become an insult, demeaning or unacceptable in modern discourse, it is placed in quote marks in first usage to indicate this, but usually not subsequently. It is important to be very clear that evidently no insult is intended when such language is used in this book; it is used solely in its historical context. We should also note that an important feature of the history of disability is the demeaning and marginalising way in which disabled people have often been characterised and addressed, and this is an aspect of the history which must be told. Issues of language are discussed in more detail in some of the discussion sections that follow each chapter. To discuss this language in the disability context is evidently hugely important and cannot be dismissed as 'political correctness' or nit-picking.

It is not straightforward, and always potentially contentious, to decide which terminology to use in a history of this nature. I have been guided as far as possible by the preferences of disability activists and the official terms used in current (2023) UK government policy. For the most part I use 'disabled people' as suggested in the social model to indicate that people are disabled by society. I use 'autistic people' as favoured by the majority of members of this community when consulted. I have however used 'people with learning disabilities', the 'people first' language favoured by many learning disability activists.

Approaches to writing a history of disability

While engaging to some extent with important issues of changing language, social attitudes, theories about disability, buildings, services and many other factors that have played an important role in shaping the life experiences of disabled people, this book also attempts to tell the individual life stories of many people who have been classified as disabled. This means not just the stories of those seen as high achievers, such as athletes and politicians who have 'overcome' their disability, but also the stories of those who have simply navigated daily life as best they can, just as most people do whether disabled or not. They might be the disabled poor begging on the streets of medieval or 18th-century London, deaf people using sign language to marry in the 16th century, or disabled veterans roaring around the countryside on adapted motorcycles after the First World War. This is ultimately a story about people and their endless adaptability and tenacity, just as much as it is a story about underlying social and economic forces which affect disability.

The book is most certainly not a medical history, although medical practitioners and institutions do play a part in it. The 'medical model' of disability is discussed within the book (p 134), in opposition to the 'social model', which was developed by disability activists in the second half of the 20th century. The medical model understands disability as a problem to be addressed or a tragedy to be alleviated through medical intervention, or otherwise managed and treated by doctors. In this model the disabled person becomes a 'patient', seen as an object of medical attention rather than an independent person with decision-making capacity. Many historians see the medical model as closely linked to, or even developing from, the religious model, which frames disability as a tragedy visited by God, and only curable by God, with the disabled person either a holy innocent or sinful. Medical histories tend to represent the story of disability as a narrative of medical progress and advance, in which disabled people only come into focus as objects of treatment.

The social model sees society as being the most prominent factor in disabling people rather than their actual impairments. Society creates physical barriers to inclusion by not adapting its spaces and buildings, but also non-physical barriers through use of language, social attitudes, lack of support and ableist assumptions. The person is not inherently 'handicapped' but is handicapped by external factors. This history draws much upon the social model but also draws upon cultural factors such as lived experience, social attitudes and interactions, the integration of disabled people into their communities in different ways at different times, and of course the self-image of disabled people. It is the story of individuals and their relations with the people and the social networks and attitudes around them – as much about how disabled people have influenced society as about how society has influenced them.

What the book covers

This book is written within a chronological framework and is divided into six time periods: medieval, 16th and 17th centuries, 18th century, 19th century, early 20th century and late 20th/early 21st century. Within each chapter several themes are covered which capture significant developments or changes in attitude identifiable in that period. These range from leprosy and the construction of hundreds of leper or lazar houses in the Middle Ages, to the construction of the great military hospitals for disabled veterans in the late 17th century, to the proliferation of small 'mad houses' in the 18th century. In more recent history, the book describes the programme of mass incarceration in asylums in the 19th century and the development of adaptive environments and technology in the later 20th century (much of which was influenced by the presence of a large newly disabled population as a consequence of the two world wars, 1914–18 and 1939–45) as well as a new focus on activism and rights.

Each chapter also aims to cover as wide a range of disabilities as possible, although it is inevitable that there will be a greater focus on certain types of disability than others in some periods, in line with differing prevailing assumptions and preoccupations at different times. While there is some concentration on buildings, because these have played a significant part in the lives of disabled people, each chapter also focuses on how disabled people have lived within their communities. The vast majority of disabled people have always lived in communities and neighbourhoods, among family, friends, neighbours and workmates. Even at the height of the 19th-century asylum era the majority did not live within institutions. This can sometimes be forgotten in accounts of disability history which are viewed through an institutional lens, driven in part by the easy availability of institutional records and the assumption that institutionalisation and disability go together.

This book is largely an English history. It arose from a web resource originally written by me for English Heritage (now Historic England) which told the disability history that lay behind and beneath many of the English buildings under its care. It makes only glancing references to developments elsewhere where these are seen as influential on the English story. Apologies are due therefore in particular to Scottish, Welsh and Irish readers, but with the good news that there is much good work elsewhere on the history of disability in their countries. Inevitably the history of England, for better or worse, is intimately and inseparably entangled with the history of the other nations that constitute Great Britain and, later, the United Kingdom. There are, however, differences in law (particularly between England and Scotland), education, and experience that justify a focus on England as a separate nation in this book, and on Scotland, Wales or Northern Ireland as separate nations in other work.

Discussion sections

At the end of each chapter there is a brief introduction to and discussion about a particular theme that is important to the understanding of the history of disability, and current and past thinking about it. These are short and very general introductions to key debates about disability and its history, aimed at informing the reader and offering a starting point for those who wish to learn and think about the issues in greater detail. This book is not a theoretical work (many readers may be relieved to hear) but the discussions point out in a broad way some of the theoretical underpinning to modern and past thinking about disability.

These discussion sections include the themes of shifting borderlands of disability, buildings, the place of special communities, charity, myths and stereotypes, models of disability, and rights and self-representation.

Sources

This history has no pretentions to consist of original research. While it does contain summaries of some elements of the author's own archival work and previous publications, it relies mainly on secondary sources from other authors, the published work of some of the small number of excellent historians who work in the field of disability history. Their work is brought together to provide an overview, and no more than that, of a thousand years of this history. All are acknowledged and readers will find a comprehensive bibliography as well as a recommended further reading list, but I would like to express my indebtedness in particular to the work of Irina Metzler and Carol Rawcliffe on the medieval period, David Turner on the 18th century, Julie Anderson on the 20th century, Jan Walmsley, Chris Goodey, Tim Stainton and Patrick McDonagh on the history of learning disability, and Tom Shakespeare on disability theory. Each of these fine historians and writers has produced pioneering work in their areas of interest, and I can only hope that I have done justice to them in the inevitably summarised versions of their findings that are now set out before the reader. Readers are highly recommended to sample their work. I am grateful also to the team at English Heritage (now Historic England), particularly Rosie Sherrington, who supported me to write the Disability in Time and Place web resource back in 2011 which inspired this book.

A glossary is provided at the end of the book to explain terms that readers, particularly those new to the subject, may be unfamiliar with.

***

Disabled people have been a part of society, influencing it and being influenced by it, throughout history. They have lived among their families and neighbourhoods, worked in fields, workshops and factories, fought in wars, played sports, begged on streets, achieved the highest office, lived both quiet and noisy lives. They have been an integral part of the complex fabric of society for as long as there has been such a thing as society. At different times they have experienced various degrees of exclusion, hostility, discrimination and oppression. They have also experienced love, integration, admiration, success, friendship and acceptance. Sometimes the lives of disabled people as a whole have progressed in a positive direction; at other times they have regressed in the face of social or political hostility. However, most of all, disabled people have made their own lives, rather than living the lives others sought to impose on them.

It is this story of complexity, variety and change that the book tells. The story is not one of unremitting progress and improvement over the centuries, and therefore it is not the story of a bad past and a good present. The 'progressive' 20th century is littered with some of the most horrendous episodes in disability history. The medieval and early modern periods, often derided as superstitious, cruel and 'primitive', have much to tell us about social adaptation and acceptance of difference. There is a great deal we can learn from the past if we can drop our condescending belief that somehow we always improve on it.

Discussion: The shifting borderlands of disability

It may seem that recognising and defining a disability is a straightforward matter. However, disability is an idea whose meaning has shifted continually through the centuries. Those who have been defined, or defined themselves, as disabled have varied significantly, just as the language used to describe what we call a disability today has changed radically over time. The implications of having a disability have also changed markedly through the centuries, and will no doubt continue to do so.

Some types of disability from the past have effectively disappeared, or can now be treated as a disease or illness without disabling consequences. Leprosy, for example, is no longer prevalent in English society. Polio, which caused widespread disability in England for much of the 20th century, has now been effectively eradicated through vaccination. Ophthalmia, which caused the blindness that affected Edward Rushton (founder of the first English Blind School in Liverpool in 1791), is now treatable (Fig 1.1).

While some conditions designated as disabilities or disabling have disappeared, other new ones have been identified. Autism, for example, was only identified during and immediately after the Second World War (1939–45). Sometimes political and social attitudes can shape what is recognised as a disability. In the first half of the 20th century the idea of the 'moral imbecile' was invented, but disappeared in the late 1950s. It was believed that moral imbeciles were people who appeared 'normal' in intelligence, but their brains lacked the capacity to understand morality, and they were therefore a danger to society. This was a disability which existed – at least in the minds of doctors and eugenicists – for just over 50 years. Many disabled activists argue that disability is just a political idea anyway – in their opinion the problem is not a person's impairment but society's disabling attitude towards people who are considered different. The shifting borderlands of disability can be a complicated matter. In this section we look in more detail at the unstable and changing meanings of leprosy, autism and moral imbecility.

Fig 1.1
The School of Industry for the Indigent Blind in Liverpool, founded by Edward Rushton. [Line engraving by H Mutlow. Wellcome Collection. Public Domain Mark]

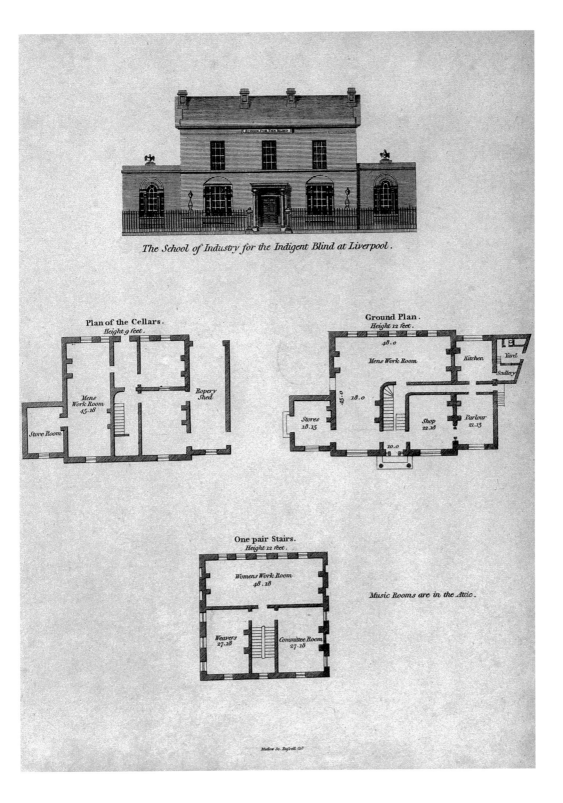

The School of Industry for the Indigent Blind at Liverpool.

Plan of the Cellars.
Height 9 feet.

Mens Work Room 45.18

Store Room

Ropery Shed

Ground Plan.
Height 12 feet.

48.0

Mens Work Room

Kitchen

Yard

Scullery

45.0   18.0

Stores 18.15

Shop 22.18

Parlour 21.13

10.0

One pair Stairs.
Height 12 feet.

Womens Work Room 48.18

Music Rooms are in the Attic.

Weavers 27.18

Committee Room 27.18

9

Leprosy

Today leprosy, now known as Hansen's disease, is not considered a necessarily disabling condition. The terms 'leper' and, to a certain extent, 'leprosy' have become offensive in modern usage, and certainly anachronistic. The disease is still prevalent in some parts of the world. However, with treatment, its disabling consequences can be avoided. Treatment also makes segregation unnecessary. When leprosy reached its peak in England in the medieval period, it was the single biggest disabling condition in the country. As a result, it caused the first big institutional response to disability – more than 300 'leper houses' or 'lazar houses' were built across England and Wales. At the end of the 14th century leprosy began to recede. It is not known why, but one theory is that it was supplanted and eradicated by the wave of bubonic plague known as the Black Death (1346–53). The leper houses were no longer needed. Some fell into disuse, but others changed their purpose. St John's Hospital in Canterbury, for example, became an almshouse. In this way leper houses laid the foundations for future institutional responses to disability such as almshouses, the madhouse, the workhouse and the asylum (Fig 1.2).

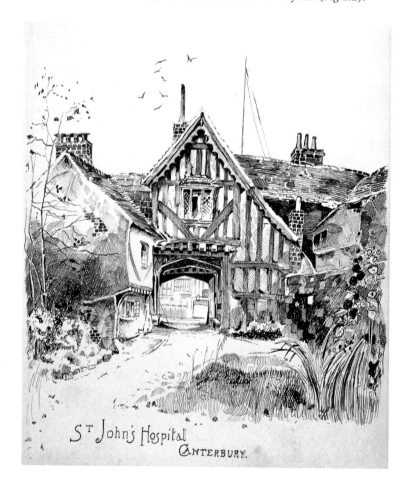

Fig 1.2
St John's Hospital Canterbury, once a leper hospital, later an almshouse.
[Drawing by E C, 1899(?). Wellcome Collection. Public Domain Mark]

St John's Hospital
Canterbury.

Nowhere reflects the shifting borderlands of disability better than the 12th-century Leper Hospital of St Mary Magdalene in Sprowston, near Norwich. Built for men with leprosy, it became a home for 'poor, aged and sick men' after the retreat of leprosy at the end of the 14th century (Fig 1.3). Today the building still stands, and more recently has been used for employment and personal development activities by people with learning disabilities. The men with leprosy for whom the building was constructed are no longer a disabled group in our society. The people with learning disabilities who have more recently used the building would not have been seen as a disabled group needing special provision in the medieval period; they would simply have lived and worked in their families and communities. Each age has its own idea of what constitutes a disability.

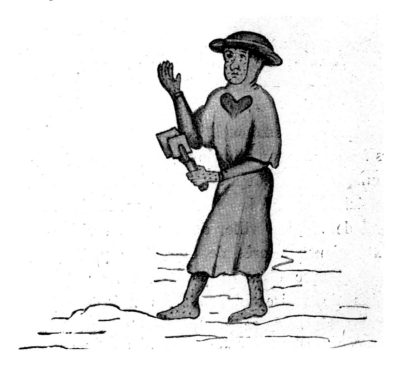

Fig 1.3
A depiction of a person with leprosy in the medieval period.
[Wellcome Collection M0001065]

Autism

The condition of autism was only identified and put forward as a form of mental disability in the 1940s by a psychiatrist and a physician working independently of each other, the American Leo Kanner (1894–1981) and the Austrian Hans Asperger (1906–80), after whom Asperger syndrome was named. Asperger has been recently discredited as a Nazi collaborator in the killing programme against disabled children during the Second World War, in research by the historian Edith Sheffer (Sheffer 2018). The attachment of his name to the condition he claimed to have identified is now controversial, and Aperger's syndrome is now being absorbed into the cluster of types of mind that are included in what we call Autism.

The relatively recent identification of autism raises interesting questions for historians of disability. Has autism always been with us, or is it a recent phenomenon? There are, of course, no historic buildings associated with autism, given that it was not even a named disability in the past. But some historians and psychiatrists have looked at case records to find past evidence of autism. In 1799, for example, a five-year-old boy at the Bethlem hospital was described in a case study. He never engaged in play with other children or became attached to them, but played in an absorbed, isolated way with toy soldiers. This is, claims one writer, possibly the first formally recorded clinical case of autism in England (Frith 1989).

Others have examined the life and work of some famous historical figures and speculated that they may have had the characteristics of autism. For example, the great scientist Sir Isaac Newton (1642–1727) was described as having a rigorously logical mind, an inability to form intimate

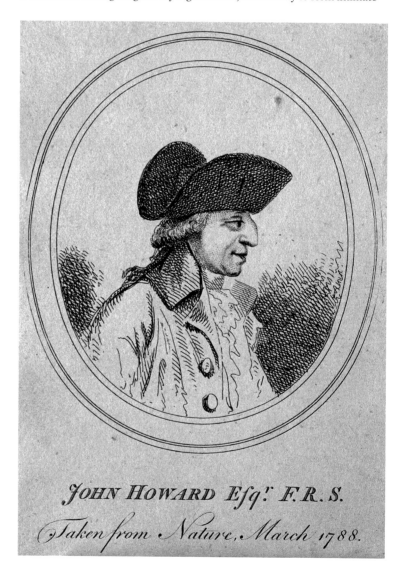

Fig 1.4
John Howard, penal reformer – characteristics of autism? [Etching 1788. Wellcome Collection. Public Domain Mark]

JOHN HOWARD Esq.ʳ F.R.S.

Taken from Nature, March 1788.

friendships, and numerous eccentric behaviours. John Howard (*c* 1726–90), the 18th-century penal reformer, travelled 60,000 miles over 17 years visiting prisons in Britain and Europe, meticulously recording and reporting everything he saw (Fig 1.4). His solitary lifestyle, intense focus on one special interest, and extreme obsession with punctuality have led to speculation that he may have had Asperger syndrome. Lewis Carroll (1832–98) (the pen name of the Reverend Charles Lutwidge Dodgson), the author of *Alice's Adventures in Wonderland* (1865), was known to have had difficulty with social interaction, narrow obsessive interests, odd speech and 'compulsive orderliness'.

However, the application of modern diagnostic criteria to historical figures can only ever be speculation. What we do know is that when Newton, Howard and Carroll were alive they may have been seen as eccentric, but were not seen as having any sort of disability or condition. They were simply valued for their extraordinary talents. Our drive to diagnose people from the past within our modern clinical categories perhaps says more about the modern urge to pathologise difference of mind than it says about individuals from the past.

'Moral imbecility'

The Mental Deficiency Act of 1913 invented as a legal entity an entirely new category of disabled person – the 'moral imbecile'. At this time proponents of the idea of eugenics were arguing that 'defective' members of the population would cause a general deterioration of the racial stock unless kept strictly controlled, segregated and, if possible, sterilised. They meant not only those who had an intellectual or physical disability, but also those they believed represented a 'moral threat' to society. These were to be found, the eugenicists believed, only in the 'lower orders' of society and could include habitual petty criminals, alcoholics, prostitutes and unmarried mothers. The meaning of 'moral imbecile' was never made entirely clear, even when in 1927 it was formally changed to 'moral defective'. It was broadly taken to mean someone who might display normal intelligence but appeared not to know the difference between right and wrong. More generally, this was identified as an amoral group whose behaviour suggested they were incapable of internalising or comprehending the moral norms of mainstream society. Thus, many people ascribed with this vague and wildly speculative deficit found themselves living in the new network of mental deficiency colonies which were built across the country, many living there until they died or not emerging until their old age.

The categories of 'moral defective' and 'moral imbecile' survived until 1959. It was therefore defined as a disability for only around half a century before being discarded. Disability in this case was nothing to do with the form of a person's body or their intellectual capacity. It was about how a person thought and behaved as perceived by others. Once more the boundaries had shifted. They will move again. 'Disability' is not a fixed idea – it changes over time and place.

2 Disability in the medieval period

Introduction and summary

Disability was pervasive in the medieval period. It could come with birth, be acquired through the onset of diseases such as leprosy, or arise from years of backbreaking work in the fields, on building sites or in workshops. The 'lepre', the 'blynde', the 'dumbe', the 'deaff', the 'natural fool', the 'idiot', the 'creple', the 'lame' and the 'lunatick' were a highly visible presence in everyday life.

Provision and support for disabled people, when it was given, came not from the state but from the Church. We see over this period the emergence of an embryonic nationwide network of early hospitals based in or near monasteries, nunneries and other religious establishments (Fig 2.1). Formed from the Christian duty of shelter to pilgrims and strangers ('hospitality'), they evolved slowly into a form of hospital caring for the sick and disabled – mostly the *poor* sick and disabled. This foreshadowed the sort of hospital we are more familiar with today. The differences between medieval hospitals and present-day hospitals are, however, as important as the similarities. They were primarily devoted to the religious life. For the small number of disabled people who lived in them, the care of their souls was given as much importance as the care or cure of their bodies. Inhabitants of the hospitals, and the almshouses which developed from the hospital idea, were mixed, comprising people with physical disabilities or sensory impairments, aged people, retired monks and nuns, lepers and others. Generally, they were people who would be destitute without the care and protection of a place of care. There was no welfare safety net outside, so when a person for some reason lacked family or friends to support them, prospects were bleak, particularly if their disability prevented them from working.

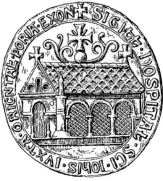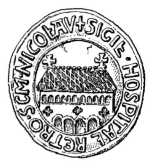

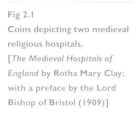

Fig 2.1
Coins depicting two medieval religious hospitals.
[*The Medieval Hospitals of England* by Rotha Mary Clay: with a preface by the Lord Bishop of Bristol (1909)]

16. HOSPITAL OF ST. JOHN, EXETER   17. HOSPITAL OF ST. ALEXIS, EXETER

We should remember, though, that despite this embryonic system of institutional care that we see develop over the period, the vast majority of disabled people, including people with mental disabilities or difficulties, lived within their families and their communities. This was where the locus of care lay. We encounter them with friends and family in groups of pilgrims visiting shrines, hoping for a saintly miracle cure which would restore their sight, their hearing, their physical functioning or their equilibrium of mind. We find them in workplaces if they were able to work. If unable to work, we see them sometimes begging on the streets. They were sometimes cared for by trade guilds when the rigours of their work had made them disabled in some way. Most of all they were cared for, if care was needed, by their families and their communities. There are many myths about disability in the medieval period. It is sometimes suggested that disabled children were killed or left to die, that disabled adults were abused, chained up or shunned. There is a belief that disabled people were outcasts because their disability was seen as a mark of sin. The truth is different. While there was some discussion about some forms or instances of disability arising from sin in some way, there was an eclectic mix of other explanations for disability, including the idea that some disabled people might be closer to God than their non-disabled fellow citizens. People were not left to die or cast out: we find them at the heart of their communities all the time, if we are only prepared to see what is in front of us. For most, such discussions were irrelevant. All they wished to do, like everyone else, was survive from day to day, and lead their everyday lives.

Buildings: early hospitals, almshouses, leper houses

The word hospital derives from the Latin word *hospes* meaning both host and guest, and is rooted in the Christian obligation to shelter any stranger, particularly passing pilgrims on their way to shrines. In the early religious establishments which provided hospitals, rules were introduced which expected the passing poor to spend one night only, but the sick were allowed to stay until they recovered, and disabled people might take up longer residence. This signalled a shift in the ethos of the hospital towards care beyond simple hospitality, foreshadowing the understanding of a hospital that we have today.

While care and support for any person with a disability throughout the medieval period remained firmly within the community, there was a steady proliferation of institutional settings that provided care. As well as hospitals there were also almshouses and leper or lazar houses. These three types of setting often overlapped or merged in both their functions and the people they served. Hospitals, almshouses and leper houses were all charitable, religiously run institutions with a spiritual ethos, focused as much on prayer and spiritual succour as on medicinal healing.

A small number of hospitals had been part of the English landscape since Anglo Saxon times. In the later Saxon period, by the 10th century the rules of St Benedict applied in English monasteries. These stipulated that hospitality should be offered to outsiders, particularly the poor and strangers; cells (small rooms) should be set aside for sick brethren who needed to be looked after; food should be provided; and alms, gifts of money or goods such as clothes should be offered. The rule of St Augustin was also influential and had spread to many religious houses with hospital functions by the end of the 15th century. This encouraged followers to lead a life of regular worship and self-discipline while carrying out charitable tasks related to the outside world, an ideal framework for the regulation of a medieval hospital (Orme and Webster 1995, 17, 70) (Fig 2.2).

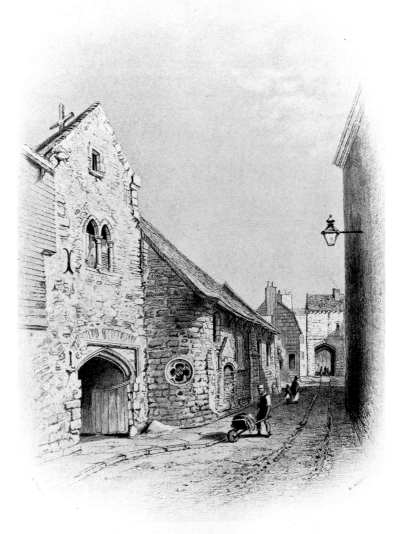

Fig 2.2
God's House Southampton, an early medieval hospital built around 1185.
[*The Medieval Hospitals of England* by Rotha Mary Clay: with a preface by the Lord Bishop of Bristol (1909)]

GOD'S HOUSE, SOUTHAMPTON

By 1080 there were an estimated 68 recorded hospital buildings in England, and over the next 500 years this increased steadily to 585 by 1530. Those who lived within these hospitals were diverse, and included lepers, poor pregnant women, the blind, the 'crippled', the insane and the epileptic (epilepsy was known as 'the falling sickness' at this time). While there is little evidence of the ailments that kept sick people under the care of these early hospitals, more is known about disabilities. At St Mary Magdalene, Ripon, in 1342, blind local priests were accommodated. In the hospital in Chatham, Kent, there were monks and nuns, some of whom were blind and one epileptic. St James' in Chichester was said to accommodate in the 16th century 'six cripples, two people without legs and two idiots' (Orme and Webster 1995, 29, 119–121). The first hospital to see its main role as the long-term care of those deemed too ill or disabled to function in wider society was St John's, Canterbury, in Kent, an early adopter of the rule of St Augustin. Established in the late 11th century by Lanfranc, the Archbishop of Canterbury, the hospital gave 24-hour care and supervision to men and women 'oppressed by various kinds of infirmities' (Clay 1909, 17, 51).

Hospitals became a feature of larger towns and cities – usually situated on the boundaries, outside the city walls rather than within. By the later Middle Ages both London and York had some 35 hospitals, Norwich 15, Exeter 10 and Canterbury 9. While some were large, such as St Mark's, Bristol, many were small, some of them little more than several cottages catering for very small groups of people. London's hospitals included St Bartholomew's, founded in 1123 under Henry I and still in existence today as the world famous Barts teaching hospital. Their position on the outskirts did not necessarily imply the marginalisation of the sick and disabled. The cleaner air outside built-up areas was regarded as good for health, and such locations offered greater opportunities to be self-sufficient in growing (and sometimes trading) food for the hospital's needs. They also lent themselves to profitable alms gathering from passing pilgrims and other travellers (Orme and Webster 1995, 41–4).

Basic layout of the larger purpose-built hospitals was quite consistent. A large 'infirmary hall' would accommodate the sick and the infirm in lines of beds to each side with a chapel in full view of all patients – the care of the soul was just as important as the care of the body (Fig 2.3). Men and women were segregated, as at the hospital of St Nicholas, Salisbury (Fig 2.4), which had two chapels linked to two infirmaries housing the two sexes (Orme and Webster 1995, 100). Caring for those with long-term disabilities was just as common as short-term or acute illnesses, and specialisms developed. For example, in 1351 St Mary within Cripplegate in London, known as 'Elsyng Spital' after its founder Elsyng, an influential London merchant, catered for 100 blind, paralytic and disabled priests (Clay 1909, 24). The word 'spital' was a derivation of the Latin *hospitale*.

For disabled people, the experience of life in an early hospital was very different from our concept of a modern hospital. They were not in any technical sense places of cure and rehabilitation, and there was little distinction between daily life in a hospital and the daily life of any house of religion (Orme and Webster 1995, 35). Hospital life centred around worship, with care of the soul its primary function. Both staff and patients

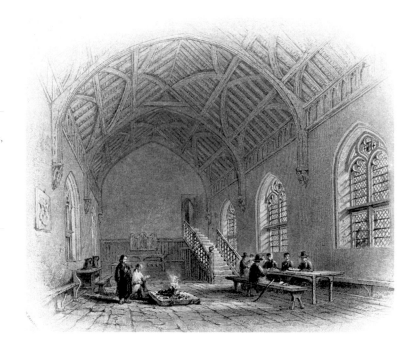

Fig 2.3
The infirmary hall of St Cross,
Winchester.
[*The Medieval Hospitals of
England* by Rotha Mary Clay:
with a preface by the Lord
Bishop of Bristol (1909)]

Fig 2.4
Hospital of St Nicholas,
Salisbury.
[*The Medieval Hospitals of
England* by Rotha Mary Clay:
with a preface by the Lord
Bishop of Bristol (1909)]

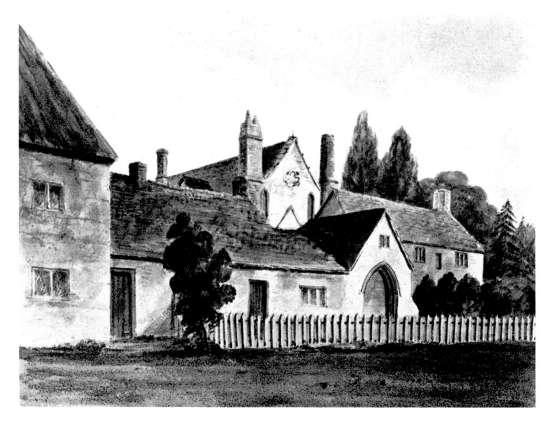

participated, and all who could rise from their beds did so and attended the chapel, up to seven times a day, on bended knees. Those who could not rise would be roused by a ringing of the infirmary bell and repeated their prayers, as well as their 200 Paternosters and Aves, sitting erect in bed (Orme and Webster 1995, 50; Clay 1909, 158–9).

Attention was also paid, of course, to bodily care, and food, fuel, baths, bedding and clothes were all provided. In a well-endowed hospital residents might get a daily loaf, a gallon of beer, meats, herring, cheese and butter. Even in poorer establishments there would often be a meat allowance of twopence a week along with vegetables and other victuals, although such establishments might be more dependent on the generosity of passing alms givers for additional food. Firewood for heating and cooking was collected with the permission of the local lord. Bedding for the sick and disabled poor consisted of pallets of straw in the early hospitals, but wooden bedsteads with coverings of animal skin were introduced from the late 12th century. There were cleanliness regimes which could involve twice-weekly head washing, bathing tubs, and hand washing before meals (Clay 1909, 167–77).

From hospitals developed the idea of the almshouse. These were sometimes referred to as a Maison Dieu, as in the Norman 'House of God', or bede house, 'bede' meaning prayer. Bede houses were founded specifically so that those who lived there could spend their lives praying gratefully for the benefactors who enabled them to do so. Almshouses were built to provide long-term shelter for disabled people and the aged infirm. They were founded and supported with donations and endowments from pious kings, church dignitaries, nobles and merchants keen to ease their passage to heaven with good works, and they became a common feature of towns and cities. Some trade guilds built almshouses for their members who could no longer sustain life in their own home. As in hospitals, there was an unrelenting regime of prayer and devotion, sustained and leavened by a decent diet and, often, pleasant gardens. There were gifts and feasts on special days. Places in almshouses were sought after, an escape from the poverty and danger that disability, old age and infirmity could bring (Bailey 1988; Hallett 2004).

Leper houses were an equally familiar feature of the English landscape, at least until leprosy's decline after the Black Death of the 1340s. At this point many former leper houses, lacking residents, became almshouses. They are discussed in more detail in the leprosy section below.

Perhaps the most famous, or infamous, of all English medieval hospitals was the priory of St Mary of Bethlehem, created in the City of London in 1247 for the healing of sick paupers. This small establishment, covering only two acres and with just 12 'cells' for patients, became known as the Bethlehem Hospital, which Londoners later abbreviated to 'Bethlem', often pronounced 'Bedlam'. At some point the monks began accepting residents whose symptoms were mental illness rather than physical disability or disease, and in this way Bethlem has come to be seen as England's first mental institution. Those taken into Bethlem tended to be the poor and destitute, sometimes viewed as dangerous, who lacked family or friends to support them. The hospital regime comprised the usual religiously inspired devotion, as attendance on and compassion

towards people afflicted by madness was a religious imperative.
However, there were also elements of corporal punishment – chains,
manacles, locks and stocks – which were believed to induce recovery in
some instances. The institution thus acquired its enduring reputation
for scandal and abuse, a reputation which intensified as it moved to
larger premises in first the17th and then the 19th century, and the word
'bedlam' entered the language, meaning a scene of uproar or confusion
(Andrews *et al* 1997, 11–129).

Yet it should be remembered that Bethlem has always occupied a
larger space in the English imagination than it ever occupied in physical
reality. As we shall see, the rightful place of the mentally ill was generally
outside institutions in the medieval period. We do see, however, in
the burgeoning network of early hospitals, almshouses, leper houses
and other buildings, the foreshadowing of the idea of the long-term
institution, set aside from mainstream society, which would later take
such a significant grip on the lives of disabled people.

The time of leprosy

Leprosy, known today as Hansen's disease, had entered England by
the 4th century and was endemic by 1050. In its extreme form it can
cause loss of fingers and toes, gangrene, blindness, collapse of the nose,
ulcerations, lesions and weakening of the skeletal frame (Fig 2.5).
Reaction to the disease in English society was complicated. It could be
seen as a punishment for sin, but it was also believed that the suffering of
lepers was similar to the suffering of Christ, thus placing them closer to
God than other people. Enduring purgatory on earth, they would ascend
directly to heaven when they died. Those who cared for them or made
charitable donations could, through these good works, accelerate their
own journey to heaven and reduce their time in purgatory.

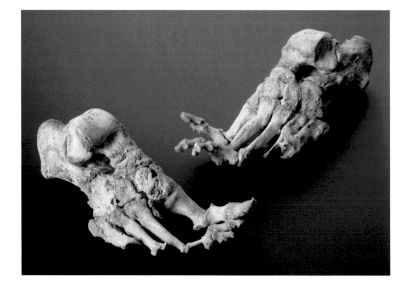

Fig 2.5
Skeletal feet of a woman with
leprosy, 14th century.
[Science Museum, London.
Attribution 4.0 International
(CC BY 4.0)]

While leprosy itself is a disease rather than a disability, it was a major cause of disability for three centuries or more. Its disabling consequences were ever more visible in communities, rural and urban, rich and poor, across England as the disease became endemic. The response would change both the landscape of the country and the mindset of its people.

An account of a 'leprous maiden' in Reginald of Durham's Miracle Collection from the early 13th century captures the range of attitudes, from malevolent to compassionate, and the role of the leper house, in the lives of people who were disabled by leprosy:

> There is a vill [equivalent to a village or parish] in the Bisopric called Hailtune in which dealt a widow and her only daughter who was greviously tormented with a most loathsome leprosy. The mother remarried a man who soon began to view the poor girl with the greatest horror, and to torment and execrate her ... She fled for aid to the priest of the vill, who, moved with compassion, procured by his entreaties the admission of the damsel to the hospital of Dernigntune [Darlington], which was almost three miles distant.
>
> (quoted in Clay 1909, 97)

The young woman remained at the hospital for three years until, in the characteristic style of miracle accounts, she was cured by St Godric, who 'removed the noxious humours', whereupon she regained her former appearance, and was pronounced fully recovered.

At least 320 religious leper houses and hospitals for the care of people with leprosy were established in England between the close of the 11th century and 1350. The prevalence of leprosy seems to have receded from around the time of the 'Black Death' in the late 1340s. There is some speculation that some form of cross immunity was caused by the plague which reduced incidence of leprosy. Many leper houses have disappeared, destroyed during the dissolution of the monasteries in the 1530s or simply decayed. However, some remain, including the oldest, St Nicholas, Harbledown, Canterbury (1070s), St Mary Magdalene, Stourbridge, near Cambridge, St Mary Magdalene in Sprowston, Norwich, and the hospital of St Mary the Virgin, Ilford. Others survive as ruins or archaeological sites.

Leper houses were usually built on the edge of towns and cities or, if they were in rural areas, near to crossroads or major travel routes. They needed to retain contact with society to beg alms, trade, and offer services such as prayers for the souls of benefactors. There was high demand for places, and 'leprous brothers and sisters' were often accepted fully into the monastic order of the house. Care from monks and nuns, as we have seen, centred as much on the person's spiritual needs as their physical problems. Most houses had their own chapel, and rituals of prayer and singing went on throughout the day. The accent was on cleanliness and wholesome food – clothes were washed twice each week and a varied diet was supplied when possible, often from the home's own fields and livestock. The therapeutic effect of horticultural work and the beauty of nature was recognised – many houses had their own fragrant gardens of flowers and healing herbs, with residents participating in their upkeep (Rawcliffe 2006).

Not all leper houses attained such standards, and when corruption or ill treatment occurred, resident lepers could show themselves not to be passive recipients of care. In 1297 the residents of the leper house in the Norfolk village of West Somerton mutinied against the embezzling prior and his men, looting and demolishing the buildings and killing the guard dog. A subsequent jury decision and court ruling supported the actions of the lepers:

> They [the jurors] said that all the lepers, before being admitted, swore an oath never to go out of the hospital, not to look over the walls, or climb trees to talk to their friends, or to complain in any way about their state, justly or unjustly … but to remain content with everything done to them without murmur or complaint. They said that no friend or stranger had access to the lepers, and that the prior had a large and strong dog tied up before the door of the hospital to prevent friends from enquiring into their condition or number, and assisting them in any necessity. Asked about the state of the house, the jurors said the chapel was roofless and very ruinous … after these disclosures the prior was ordered to maintain, for nothing, the poorest and neediest lepers as the manor would support, to repair and maintain the buildings, not to exact an oath in future, and to absolve those who had taken one.
>
> (quoted in Rawcliffe 2006, 317–8)

Lepers, like other disabled people, made pilgrimages with friends and family to holy sites such as the shrine of Thomas Becket in Canterbury, in search of a cure or at least relief. Many of them chose to live outside institutions, or could not gain places in them. Groups lived in small informal settlements just outside or even sometimes within towns (Fig 2.6). Some remained in their homes, cared for by their families and visited by monks and clergy. Margery Kempe, a 15th-century mystic from Kings Lynn, observed that the many lepers in the streets reminded her of Christ 'with hys wowndys bleeding'. Kempe demonstrated Christian compassion towards lepers, and defied fear of contagion by kneeling and kissing two leprous women 'for the love of Ihesu [Jesus]' (Rawcliffe 2006, 129, 290). Governments and municipalities, fearful of a rebellious underclass and wary of 'wild' lepers (as opposed to the supposedly more 'docile' sort who lived in leper houses) issued edicts to try to control the problem. Permits for begging were strictly controlled, and in 1367 the London authorities tried to impose a blanket ban on lepers entering the city (Rawcliffe 2006, 289) (Fig 2.7).

Many in leper houses retained their contacts with their family and friends, being allowed to make visits home and to receive visitors. Attitudes began to change in the 14th century, particularly after the horrors of the Black Death (1347–50), as fear of contagion led to greater restriction and isolation. At the same time, abusive and corrupt practices increased. However, by this time leprosy was in retreat and many houses fell into disuse or were put to new uses, such as St Mary Magdalene, Ripon, and St Margaret and St Sepulchre, Gloucester, which became almshouses for the sick and disabled poor. The impact of leprosy lived on – it had brought about an institutional response to disablement in the form of buildings and methods of care which would strongly influence future thinking about disability.

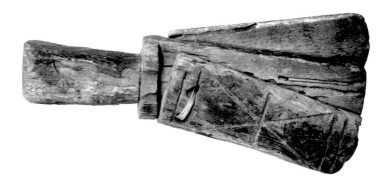

Fig 2.6
Leper clappers were used to denote the presence of lepers, and also to draw attention for begging purposes.
[Wellcome Collection. Attribution 4.0 International (CC by 4.0)]

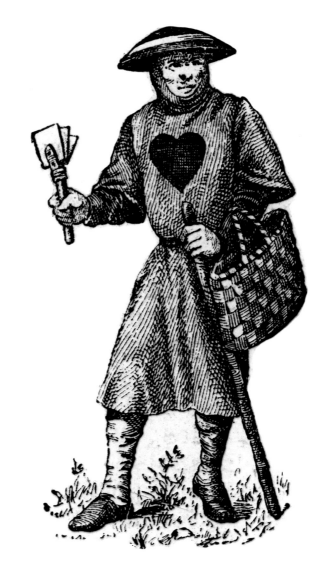

Fig 2.7
Many lepers chose to live outside institutions.
[Wellcome Collection. Attribution 4.0 International (CC by 4.0)]

Physical and sensory impairment

Opinions about the causes of physical and sensory impairment, and attitudes towards disabled people, were diverse and variable in the Middle Ages. There was a belief that disability could be caused by sin, but this did not apply to all cases. A Church decree of 1215, which soon became part of Canon Law across Europe, stated that 'since bodily infirmity is sometimes caused by sin … physicians should ensure that patients hear confession before medical treatment is applied, so that the soul could be cured prior to the body' (Metzler 2006, 47). The implication that physical disability was not always caused by sin was clear. There was a widespread acceptance that destitution, deformity and degeneration were normal phenomena associated with the human condition following the fall and original sin of mankind.

The body was also seen as a microcosm of the wider cosmos, in other words a miniature, mirror version of the world outside it. Just as in the wider world imbalance and corruption could undermine good order, illness and disability could impact on the balance and stability of an individual's body and mind. Impairment could even be seen as bringing a person closer to God, as confinement caused by arthritis, paralysis or other forms of immobility would ensure that a person pursued interior contemplation over an active life, and thus increase their holiness. As with other forms of bodily or mental affliction, physical and spiritual healing were often accorded equal standing (Metzler 2006, 45–8).

The imbalance that impairment or deformity were thought to bring, however, was not generally regarded as positive. Harmony was seen as beauty and therefore a lack of harmony, symmetry or proportion in a human body could be seen as correspondingly ugly. Thomas Aquinas wrote, 'there are two kinds of deformity in the human body. In one there is a defect in some limb, so that we call mutilated people ugly. What is missing in them is a due proportion [of parts] to the whole.' This lack of completeness, to Aquinas, meant that disabled people were 'deficient in certain symmetries and correspondences' (quoted in Metzler 2006, 51). In this way the presence of disabled people could be woven into the fabric of the deepest fear of the period, social disorder and imbalance.

For most people with physical or sensory impairment throughout the Middle Ages, such rarefied intellectual musings had little impact on their daily lives. Their task was to get through each day. Those who could worked, often with levels of disability that would be seen by many as precluding them from the workplace in modern societies. Tasks such as gleaning (collecting ears of corn after the bulk of a harvest had been brought in) could be assigned to disabled people, as well as the elderly and children, as it was less physically demanding than other harvest tasks such as reaping. However, such work would only be assigned if a person's disability incapacitated them from harder labour. Whatever a person's impairment, if they could carry out the more difficult and arduous tasks they would be expected to do so (Metzler 2013, 78).

Those who could not work relied on support from family. Beyond that the proceeds of begging were their best option (Fig 2.8). A very small proportion of the population of disabled people, as we have seen, were accommodated in early hospitals or almshouses, all of them provided

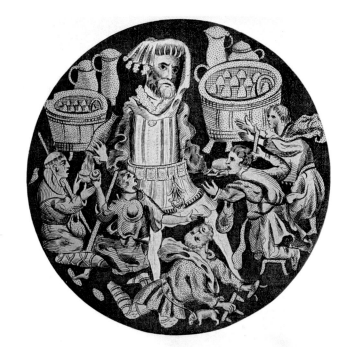

THE BEGGARS' DOLE

Fig 2.8
The Beggar's Dole – note
the stool support and hand
crutches used by disabled
beggars.
[*The Medieval Hospitals of
England* by Rotha Mary Clay:
with a preface by the Lord
Bishop of Bristol (1909)]

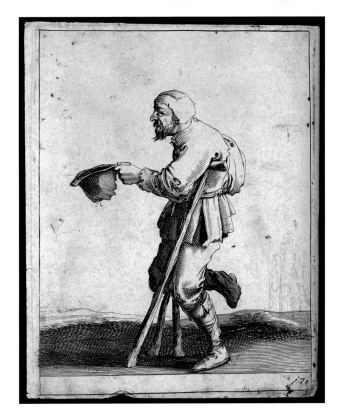

Fig 2.9
A disabled beggar seeks alms
in the medieval period.
[Engraving with etching.
Wellcome Collection. Public
Domain Mark]

by religious orders. Outside the institutions beggars were omnipresent, not only in towns but also on country roads, outside churches and in marketplaces. As well as those who were simply destitute through economic circumstances, the ranks of beggars included particular groups such as widows, orphans and the physically impaired. Physical impairment comprised the 'crippled', the lame and the blind. The non-disabled were encouraged to give alms to beggars, particularly disabled beggars, while in good health, to demonstrate piety, worthiness and virtue (Metzler 2013, 164) (Fig 2.9).

Work accidents were often the cause of long-term disability. Saint Walstan, who had a shrine in Norfolk, came to be seen as a saint who could cure impairments, enabling a return to employment. This was important because an inability to work as the result of a disabling accident could presage destitution. His miracles included the cure of a lame weaver, and of a carter who had been crushed during harvest time, both of whom rushed back to their work having received miraculous intervention at the saint's shrine (Metzler 2013, 44).

Because the consequences of disability could be so impoverishing, trade guilds would seek to support members who became disabled and were no longer able to pursue their trade. The guild of tailors in Norwich provided a penny a day for members who had become disabled, particularly those with back problems or blindness, caused by the poor light and cramped conditions in which they worked. The Guild in Hull, from the mid-14th century, gave sevenpence a week to those who became 'infirm, bowed, blind, deaf, maimed or sick … whether in old age or youth' (Metzler 2013, 62).

Miracle narratives recount the saintly cures of the whole range of disabilities. In 1173 St Bartholomew was said to have cured a young woman who was deaf, dumb, blind and crippled. Brought by her parents to the festival of St Bartholomew, she regained her sight, hearing, and mobility, whereupon she went 'joyfull skipping forth … [and] ran to the table of the holy awter [altar] spredyng out both hands to heuyn [heaven] and so she that a litill before was dum joynyg in laude [praise] of God perfitly sowdynd her wordes'. After this she wept with joy at her liberation. Many other miracle tales portrayed similar events, where the blind could see again and the deaf could hear, paralysed youths were slowly able to move once more, or workers regained the use of crippled hands (Clay 1909, 95–6) (Fig 2.10).

Such stories attest to the central role of religion in understandings of disability in the medieval period. Impairment came from God and, logically, could only therefore be removed by God, usually through the works of divine saintly representatives. To our modern eyes such miraculous cures might lend themselves to the rational explanations we crave, such as natural restoration of bodily functioning over a time after an accident given a divine explanation, or simply as fantasies expressing yearning for the removal of a person's disability. Whatever the function of these accounts, they reveal the parity of care of the soul with care of the body in medieval thought, and it was in this context that bodily impairment was understood. The person with a disability, like everyone else, was in the hands of God and at the mercy of God. Alongside this religious mindset sat a very secular and practical determination to get on

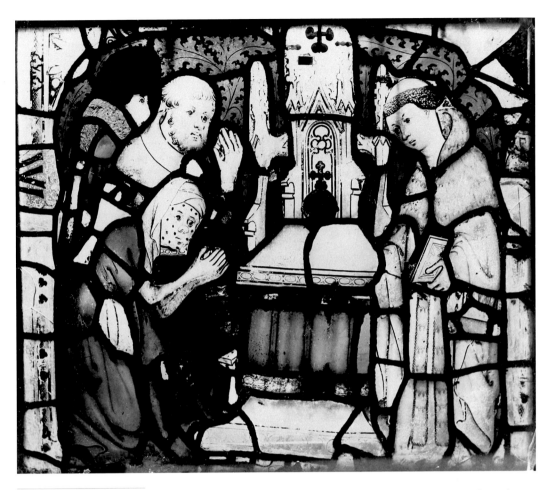

Fig 2.10
Miracle accounts show how disabled people sought cure through saintly intervention. Leper woman praying at the shrine of St William, window at York Minster.
[Wellcome Collection. Attribution 4.0 International (CC by 4.0)]

with life, through work if possible, and, for the vast majority of people, within their family and their community. The disabled person was at the heart of the social nexus, and was not an exotic curiosity or outcast.

Mental illness

How were people understood in the Middle Ages who had what we would call today a mental illness or mental health condition, and who in the past have been designated as 'mad' or 'lunatic'? During this period intellectuals, including practitioners of medicine, and ordinary people were acutely aware of different types of mental health condition. People could be described as insane or possessed, mad, furious, frantic, alienated, confused, foolish, frenzied or demonically possessed. It was broadly accepted that mental disturbance, as with most other ailments, derived from an imbalance of the four humours in the brain, which were in Latin *phrenitis* (frenzy), *lethargos* (lethargy), *mania* (mania) and *melancholia* (melancholy) (Trenery 2019, 9–10). An overabundance of any one of those humours would determine the type of mental disturbance a person would suffer from. Too much melancholy or lethargy would result in depressive-type behaviour, while too much mania or frenzy could result in manic or violent episodes. Cure could be effected by restoring the balance of the humours.

We can glean much about medieval attitudes towards mental disturbance through the enormously popular miracle accounts, written mostly by monks, and consisting of 'hagiographies', or biographies of saints with accounts of the miracles that were attributed to them. Miracle accounts contained both supernatural and natural explanations of mental disturbance, and such disturbance could be understood as having religious, magical, natural, demonic and medical causes, sometimes simultaneously. There was no sharp division between medical and magical explanations or solutions. Science and the supernatural were not separate modes of thought, but often combined.

Madness could be seen as a punishment from God. In the late 11th-century miracles of St Edmund the Martyr in Bury (now Bury St Edmunds), those who disrespected the saint in some way could be driven out of their senses, possessed by demons or forced into frenzies for their transgression. In one account, a Dane called Osgood approached St Edmund's tomb while drunk and went to lean irreverently on his axe. God caused the axe to be thrown against the wall, and Osgood fell to the floor in a frenzy. The monks prayed for Osgood's reconciliation with the saint and he recovered his senses, although he lost his sense of touch in his hands, which was a permanent reminder of his sin (Trenery 2019, 29). The punishment of madness in this case, with its very physical manifestations as a warning to others, was divine, and so was the mercy that cured it.

In Thomas Monmouth's *Life and Miracles of William of Norwich* (1154–55) madness was seen as an illness more than a punishment, although in Williams's cult there was much violence in the miracle accounts, which often involved a high level of physical restraint. Sufferers who were eventually cured by William broke their chains, tried to bite and scratch bystanders, shook, had seizures, self-harmed and sometimes had to be restrained by several men. A man called Ebrard Fisher was 'vexed by an unclean spirit', which resulted in him attacking people, blaspheming and trying to bite and scratch. His hands were tied behind his back, his feet were bound, and a group of men brought him to William's tomb. Saint William cured him, and he became quiet, able to sleep and eat, healthy and joyful (Trenery 2019, 64). In this case, Ebrard Fisher was not being punished for anything. His mental disturbance had natural causes, but his cure was divine. It is possible that the violence inherent in William's miracles derived from the origins of his sanctification. The story of William of Norwich is infamous as the world's first written blood libel against a Jewish community. The Jews of Norwich were falsely accused of violently and ritually murdering William, a local Christian boy.

The most famous cult of this period, that of Thomas Becket in Canterbury, combined both the latest medical knowledge of the time and enduring notions of demonic possession in its explanations of madness. Becket, the Archbishop of Canterbury, was murdered in Canterbury Cathedral in 1170. Miracles started to occur within days of his death and a large cult quickly grew centred on his shrine in the cathedral.

The compilers of these miracles, William of Canterbury and Benedict of Peterborough, were custodians of the shrine and are known to have asked questions of recipients of cures about both sickness and healing (Trenery 2019, 83).

The miracle accounts of the Becket cult differ from their predecessors in their highly detailed records of people's conditions and their focus on the causes of their illnesses, which suggests that both compilers had access to 'new' (in the sense that they were new to Britain) medical texts in their monasteries and were applying some of this knowledge alongside traditional demonic explications for madness (Trenery 2019, 85). For example, William Patrick is described as having 'a tumour that caused him excruciating toothache. Because of the pain, he flung his limbs and shouted out. Under suspicion he was mad, he was put in chains. Becket later cured his tumour' (Trenery 2019, 87). There is a naturalistic explanation of the cause of his madness, but a religious cure.

Another miracle describes Matilda of Cologne, who came to Becket's shrine in Canterbury 'suffering from insanity', tearing her smock and striking out at people, including a small child. During several hours at Becket's tomb she was visited by the saint in a vision, who told her to continue her pilgrimage, and after this she was cured. She told the monks when questioned after her cure that her madness had been caused by her brother killing her lover, after which she had attacked and killed her baby. Just as William Patrick's madness was explained by his physical pain, so Matilda of Cologne's insanity was attributed to her quite rational torment at the traumas that had occurred in her life.

However, in the same miracle collection, accounts were given of people whose madness was caused by demonic possession. An illegitimate Frenchman called Hugh Brustins was 'possessed by an impure spirit', but after being told that a new saint (Becket) was performing cures, he was healed with water infused with Becket's blood. A servant called Robert was 'taken by a demon, which took control of his hands', but he too was cured by drinking the martyr's blood, although he had to do this twice as the result of a relapse. In Essex two 'possessed women' were cured by drinking the holy water of St Thomas (Trenery 2019, 88–9). As well as demonic possession, divine punishment could also be a factor. A man called Ralph Black, who had dissuaded his shipmates from making a pilgrimage to Canterbury, was inflicted with madness as a result. He was bound with rope to contain his fighting, and his 'roving eyes filled with fire'. He was only restored to soundness of mind after making a vow to the martyr Thomas.

In the cult of St Thomas, madness could be caused by both physical or mental factors, or be the result of divine punishment or demonic possession. Religious and medical explanations could sit comfortably intermingled in the medieval mind both as the causes and cures of insanity.

In the miracles of Saint Hugh of Lincoln, who died in 1197 and was canonised in 1220, there is one particularly fascinating miracle narrative, occurring during Hugh's lifetime, that holds both demonic and naturalistic explanation simultaneously and without contradiction. A madman consumed by acute fever had to be restrained by eight sane men to stop him from devouring his wife and children. Hugh

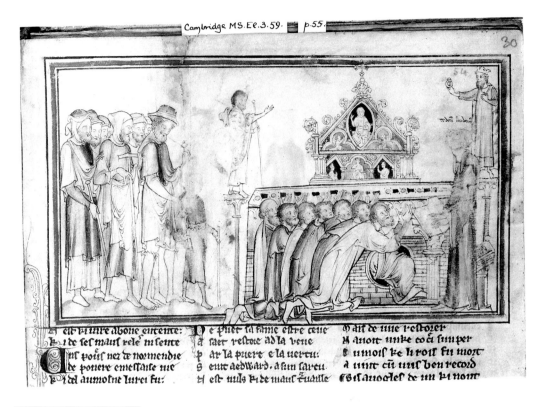

Fig 2.11
Miracles at the tomb of
Edward the Confessor.
[Wellcome Collection.
Attribution 4.0 International
(CC by 4.0)]

used holy water to exorcise and cure him. The miracle narrative gives
a naturalistic, medicalised account of the cold water acting against
the madman's hot blood and cooling both his body and his madness,
but also juxtaposes the effect of holy water against the unholy demon,
resulting in the demon's expulsion. Both the cure and the madness
were simultaneously spiritual and physical. This was certainly not a
medicalised explanation of 'madness' as we would understand it today
(Trenery 2019, 148).

There was then, across the medieval period, an understanding
of the concept of the disordered, imbalanced or irrational mind, and
its potential curability. Understandings of the causes of such mental
afflictions, how they could be treated or cured, and the implications for
people who endured them, varied considerably, not only over time but
between places. It was certainly not the case that mental illness was seen
solely as a punishment from God for some form of sin, nor was it given the
more materialist explanations rooted in brain dysfunction that dominate
21st-century medicine. Naturalistic, scientific, supernatural and religious
explanations were intermixed. A single episode of mental imbalance
might have a supernatural cause, such as a demon, and a natural cure,
such as water. Similarly, an episode could be seen as arising from natural
causes such as a tumour but be cured miraculously by saintly intervention.
The borderland between science and religion in understanding mental
imbalance was highly permeable, and was often not recognisable as a
borderland at all.

Most notable from the miracle accounts is that people seen as mentally ill were not confined to institutions. They lived their lives in their communities, and however problematic their condition became, it was friends, neighbours and families who would accompany them to shrines and seek cure for them. The natural place for care when it was needed was the community, not the institution and, as we have seen, the number of 'mad' people detained in the very few institutions that existed, such as Bedlam, was tiny. Responses were sometimes brutal to modern eyes, with people tied by their hands and feet if they were deemed to be dangerous or out of control. But the focus of communities was generally on cure and protection rather than punishment or ostracisation.

'Idiocy'

In 1290 the English patent rolls, an administrative record expressing the king's will on a wide range of matters of public interest, contained the following brief summary:

> Appointment of Juliana, mother of Henry son of John de Holewell, to the custody of his body and lands in the County of Hertford, as it appears by the inquisition before Ralph de Hengham and his fellows, justices of the King's Bench, that he has been an idiot from his birth.
>
> (quoted in Metzler 2016, 168)

Throughout the medieval period there was a recognition of a lifelong mental condition of low mental faculty which, unlike mental illness, was characteristic of a person from birth, and could affect their capacity to function in society. This group fell under the broad category of 'idiots', which was a far more neutral description in the Middle Ages than the term of abuse it has become today.

Social and legal recognition of such a condition, which was carefully distinguished from mental illness, had existed since antiquity. In early Greek society the word *idiota* signified a private person, with the implication that they did not participate, or lacked the capacity to participate, in public life. Both the word and the idea passed into English law, with the requirement that those deemed idiotic through lack of judgement or comprehension should be made wards. This meant that they should be looked after, and their affairs managed, either by their families or their lords. Such wardship became the responsibility of the monarch in England in the late 13th century, in the time of Edward I, as part of the Prerogativa Regis (Prerogative of the King), a document which asserted the rights of the crown over those considered to lack mental capacity (Metzler 2016, 47; Jarrett 2020, 23–4).

The term idiocy carried a number of meanings. It could mean simply an uneducated, ignorant person, and for the small, educated elite of this period that description applied to most people. In this sense it could mean 'stupid peasant', an idea of rural simplicity and dull-wittedness that has persisted ever since. However, it could have a more specific meaning of a person with a more marked deficiency in mental capacity who might struggle to understand the basics of everyday life (Metzler 2016, 45,

205–6). Other terms were used that attempted to capture the complexity of different levels of mental ability, such as the Latin *hebes* (dull-witted), *fatuus* and *stultus* (foolish or stupid) (Metzler 2016, 37–8). A common term to describe the person seen as lacking mental faculty was 'natural fool'. This indicated that the person was born this way and would always remain so. Idiocy was their natural (and so in that sense God-given) condition.

Although understandings of idiocy changed and developed from the early to late Middle Ages, certain characteristics were commonly ascribed to the so-called idiotic person. These included an inability to form judgements and understand abstract concepts, difficulties in speech and communication, perpetual childishness, idiosyncratic behaviours, deficiencies of memory, problems in managing responsibilities, and self-neglect (Metzler 2016, 115, 119, 122; Turner 2018, 27, 34). There was also a belief that idiots had a particular appearance, such as small or pointy heads (Metzler 2016, 223). Konrad of Magdeburg wrote in his *Book of Nature* in the 14th century:

> The person of a stupid nature is either very pale or coloured very dark, has a fat belly and bent fingers. His face is round and very fleshy. But also he is stupid whose neck and feet, in fact whose whole body, is very fleshy. His belly is round and protruding. His shoulders drawn up toward the head. His forehead is round as a bull, humped and fleshy. His jaws are strongly developed and his legs long.
>
> (quoted in Metzler 2016, 73)

Idiocy, because of its incurable, unchanging nature, was of no interest to medical practitioners, whose trade depended on the ability to cure and make better. There was a general absence of idiocy as a subject in medical textbooks of the period. Without medical interest, the responsibility for care for the idiot person remained with the family and the community, and the number of idiots who found themselves in medieval hospital institutions such as Bethlem was remarkably small. Nor was idiocy seen as a particularly religious matter. Being natural – and therefore determined by God – idiocy was not generally seen as a mark of sin. If it was not a sin, then a cognitive deficit could not be cured by a miracle, and so the appearance of idiots in miracle healings was extremely rare (Metzler 2016, 58, 84, 228).

Neither pathologised by doctors, nor ensnared in divine explanations, overwhelmingly idiocy was perceived as a practical matter, related to a person's ability to function in society. Those who might be diagnosed as having a mild or moderate learning disability in our modern societies today were simply able to get on with it in a society where most people were illiterate and the ability to 'get by' was the main prerequisite of daily life. Legal inquisitions to determine idiocy under Prerogativa Regis therefore tested whether a person's responsibilities were being neglected, and if they were capable of carrying them out. Self-neglect or property neglect were important indicators of whether a person could rule their own lands or their own self (Turner 2018, 27–8, 33–4). This was of great importance in matters such as the management of land and estates, and there was therefore a significant class element in whether or not it mattered if a person was an idiot. If they owned property or land, were in a position to sell or bequeath it, or were likely to inherit it, then their capabilities and their potential vulnerability to exploitation were important. The maintenance of noble bloodlines also mattered, and inappropriate or exploitative marriage contracts could raise issues of capacity. For landless peasants who had nothing to bequeath or inherit, however, the vulnerabilities of idiocy were a matter nor for the courts but for the family or local community.

Crown officials who carried out hearings to determine idiocy never drew on medical or religious expertise. They simply carried out pragmatic 'tests' which would enable a common-sense determination. People would be asked questions about the names of their relatives, where they lived, or where the court was taking place, and also practical questions about dates, weights and measures, and coinage (Turner 2018, 31). Records of hearings showed that conclusions were drawn from the answers people gave to such questions about their capacity for self-determination, and whether they needed to be put into the hands of a guardian or 'keeper'.

Records of a number of such cases survive. John Byrt, for example, was described as 'an idiot from birth, unable to manage himself or his lands', while John Harpesfield 'was an idiot from birth with insufficient sense to manage his lands and tenements'. A woman called Emma Beston was deemed not to have 'the intelligence to manage herself, her lands or her goods' after she was unable to answer questions on the name of her former husbands, how many shillings there were in 40 pence and the names of the days of the week. While it is not always possible to determine whether the people questioned in these hearing were born 'natural fools' or had somehow acquired their lack of mental faculty, there was a clear medieval distinction between an incurable cognitive impairment of some sort and a curable episode of mental illness (Turner 2018, 33; Metzler 2016, 163–4).

The idiot was a person clearly recognised in medieval society, their potential weaknesses and vulnerabilities understood, but their place solidly within the communities into which they were born.

Conclusion

As we have seen, disability in the medieval period was a community matter, and the families and communities of England were accepting of, and adapted to, disability in their midst. For most, life was tough and precarious, and destitution through loss of work or the ability to work, loss of family and neighbourhood support, or the acquisition of a disabling disease such as leprosy could always be sensed lurking just around the corner.

Judgement of disability could be harsh. It could be characterised as a mark of sin, as contagious, as 'ugly' or as an indicator of spiritual or moral degeneration. The opposite was also true. Disabled people could be seen as close to God through their suffering, reminiscent of the suffering of Christ (Fig 2.12). They could be the object of love, support and devotion from those closest to them, simply through being a family member or

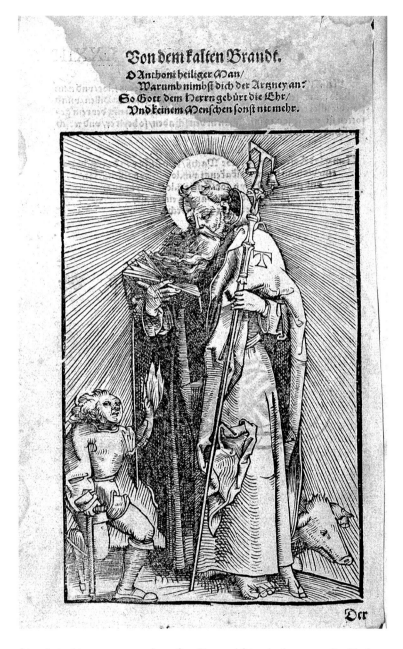

Von dem kalten Brandt.

O Anthoni heiliger Man/
Warumb nimbst dich der Artzney an?
So Gott dem Herrn gebürt die Ehr/
Vnd keinem Menschen sonst nit mehr.

friend. And it was among those families and friends that most disabled
people lived.

The people, towns and cities of the medieval period, and in particular
their religious orders, pioneered the use of specialist buildings and a form
of professional organisation in response to disability. While most disabled
people remained outside the orbit of these new structures, they were an
important foundation stone in the development of public and charitable
services that would unfurl over the following 500 years.

Discussion: Buildings and the history of disability

The medieval period saw the first use of specialist buildings for the care of disabled people. This section discusses the place of the special building in the history of disability, and the legacy of medieval approaches.

Can we say that in some way the history of disability is about the history of buildings? It can be tempting to see it that way. Specialist buildings, either in their design or their function, have played a significant part in the lives of disabled people throughout history. The medieval period had its monastery hospitals, leper houses and almshouses that were seen as the fulfilment of the religious duty to care for and provide 'hospitality' to those who could not care for themselves. In the 16th and 17th centuries in England, after the dissolution of Catholic monasteries and seizure of their buildings, buildings with a more secular ethos appeared, such as the grand military hospitals for wounded and disabled sailors and soldiers in Greenwich and Chelsea. The 18th century gave us small madhouses, the first deaf and blind schools, and more specialist hospitals, such as Guy's in London. The 19th century produced a huge expansion of disability-focused building in the form of asylums, workhouses and schools. Throughout the 20th century buildings were constructed or adapted for disability use – colonies for the 'defective', homes and facilities for disabled war veterans, specialist workplaces, residential homes, day centres, adaptive housing and so on.

However, it is important to note that the role that buildings have played in the lives of disabled people has often been controversial. Some viewed the asylums of the 19th century as places of safety for vulnerable people. Others, at the time and since, have seen them as places of incarceration to exclude people from society – 'convenient places for inconvenient people' as one historian has described them. 'Madhouses' could be seen by the public in the 18th century both as places of humanity and recuperation for people suffering mental illness and as abusive institutions for locking away unwanted family members.

Given the important role they have played, it is therefore possible to tell a history of disability through buildings over a 1,000-year period. However, to do so would be to risk telling only a partial history, and one which will distort the true history of the lived experience of disabled people. As is highlighted throughout this book, the majority of disabled people have always lived outside specialist buildings, within their communities, even at the height of the institution in the 19th century.

In the medieval and early modern (16th to 18th centuries) periods, through to the beginning of the 19th century, care and support were almost exclusively local. The average disabled person, like most people, invariably lived within a few miles of where they were born for their whole lives. On the streets of large cities, disabled people jostled for position with everyone else. Some begged, many worked, and where their disabilities caused them problems in participating in daily life, they adapted as best they could. Creative mobility technologies were produced, such as wooden curved 'bowls' in which legless people could sit and propel themselves using small hand crutches. Sticks, crutches, artificial legs and other walking aids were ingeniously constructed from any wood that was to hand. Blind people were guided by dogs, children or relatives. Deaf people used 'ear trumpets', lip reading or sign language to communicate.

Institutions, specialist buildings, were only ever for the few. They were neither the lucky few nor the unlucky few. A combination of factors took them into buildings. Sometimes they were monks or nuns who had become disabled in some way and were simply looked after by their own communities. Others were disabled people who had become destitute and had lost any form of family or friendship network – it was the combination of disability and destitution, not disability in its own right, that propelled them into an institution or specialist building of some sort. People with leprosy found themselves in specialist leper houses in part because of a fear of contagion, but also because the clean air and pleasing views that were a feature of many of these buildings offered them a chance of the recuperation, tranquillity and spirituality thought to be the best treatment for their condition. They moved in and out between these buildings, while many, known as 'wild lepers', chose not to live in such buildings at all. Institutions were not seen at this time as obligatory, and institutionalisation for disabled people was far from the norm. Indeed, it was far from possible for most.

During the 19th century the special building began to be seen far more as the 'correct' destination for disabled people, the expectation of care shifting from the community to the institution. There were deep-seated changes in attitude across the ideological spectrum. After the French Revolution of 1789, left-wing idealists found no space for the disabled citizen in the utopian new societies they wished to build. Conservatives feared difference as a driver of revolution and social turmoil, and sought to construct what they saw as a more conforming, orderly society based on ideas of what constituted 'normality'. All of this was coupled with the rise of a growing bureaucratic state that intervened in the lives of its citizens far more than had been the case previously. If you did not 'fit in', you were relocated from society and put somewhere seen as more appropriate for you – a building, and usually a place, which separated you from the rest of society, and family and community life. Such attitudes can linger on today, despite the closure of many of the large institutions in the final decades of the 20th century. A 'specialist service' is still seen by many as the 'right' destination for a disabled person (Fig 2.13).

One danger that lurks in telling the history of disability as a history of buildings is that it accepts this 19th- and 20th-century notion that the specialist building is where a disabled person belongs – the disabled person is in effect a 'creature of the institution'. The relationship between disabled people and buildings, and how the building can shape negative images of disability, has been explored by some theorists. In 1961, for example, the American sociologist Erving Goffman published his book *Asylums: Essays on the Social Situation of Mental Patients and other Inmates* (Fig 2.14). He argued that incarceration in an institution caused the mentally or physically disabled person to suffer what he called a 'civil death', in which dispossession of rights and the ability to participate in the wider world become inevitable and irrevocable. In such institutions the sense of time and purpose is lost, and the person becomes disconnected from hope, meaning and the social

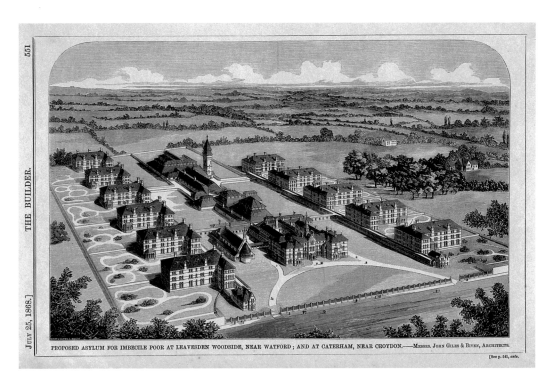

551

THE BUILDER.

JULY 25, 1868.]

PROPOSED ASYLUM FOR IMBECILE POOR AT LEAVESDEN WOODSIDE, NEAR WATFORD; AND AT CATERHAM, NEAR CROYDON.——MESSRS. JOHN GILES & BIVEN, ARCHITECTS.

[See p. 541, ante.

Fig 2.13
Separated from society:
design for Leavesden and
Caterham imbecile asylums,
near London, 1870.
[Wood engraving by W C
Smith, 1868, after J Giles &
Bivan. Wellcome Collection.
Public Domain Mark]

connectedness that most others enjoy to some extent in their lives (Goffman 1961).

In 1975 another theorist, Wolf Wolfensberger, argued that the institution inevitably degraded the perception and self-esteem of disabled people. Writing in particular about those he called 'the retarded', he said that within such buildings people became dehumanised through being characterised as sick, subhuman or a menace. Further, he argued, even in buildings constructed with ostensibly humane and positive intentions, the person could only become an object of pity, burden of charity, or be seen as some sort of disconnected 'holy innocent'. According to Wolfensberger each of these perceptions is just as dehumanising as more overtly negative perceptions such as the menace or the subhuman (Wolfensberger 1975). The institutional building, both Goffman and Wolfensberger argued, is intimately connected with the negative construction of the idea of disability and the dehumanisation of the person perceived as disabled.

Not everyone agrees with Wolfensberger's and Goffman's assertion that specialist buildings are *necessarily* and *inevitably* institutional, dehumanising and oppressive. The sociologist and activist Tom Shakespeare accepts that institutions such as schools, long-stay hospitals, clinics and workplaces are places where labels and meanings of disability 'can be concocted'. However, he points out that even if none of these institutions existed, disability would still exist. The 85 per cent of the disabled population of the world who do not get access to services would probably, he adds, willingly accept a bit of 'governmentality', the word used by critics of institutional services to describe state interventions and support systems (Shakespeare 2014, 66–7).

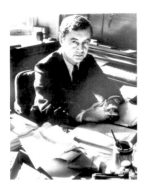

Fig 2.14
Erving Goffman (1922–82).
[American Sociological
Association]

The case has been made by the medieval historian Carol Rawcliffe that leper houses, despite their poor historical reputation, could be enlightened havens of kindness and closely connected to their communities. The great military hospitals of the 17th and 18th centuries certainly seemed to offer a better life to disabled war veterans than begging on the streets, as had often been their lot previously. Yet incidents of institutional abuse and cruelty litter history, and they continue in our societies today.

There are therefore two important conclusions to draw from this discussion. First, the history of disability is not the history of disability-related buildings, although these buildings do play a significant part in the history. Building-centred histories of disability must always be understood in relation to their opposite, the millions of disabled people throughout history who never went anywhere near a specialist building in their lives. Disability in history is embedded both within communities and within separated buildings and spaces.

Second, the history of disability-related buildings is itself complex, and can be a mix of good and malevolent intentions, of institutional abuse and havens of kindness, creativity or positivity. Such buildings are always to a large extent the product of the social mores and cultural attitudes of their time.

3 Dissolving and reforming: Tudors and Stuarts, 1485–1714

Introduction and summary

The great changes that occurred in English society in the 16th century had a marked effect on the lives of disabled people. Henry VIII's dissolution of the monasteries in the 1530s, an assault on the buildings and other assets of the Catholic religious orders after his split from the Roman Catholic Church, caught up in its wake many hospitals and places of care that were run by religious brethren. As these disappeared, so did the systems of care that went with them. For those with disabilities who had lived in these places, this meant destitution and life on the streets. A petition to Henry in 1538 from the Lord Mayor of London, Richard Gresham, calling for the refoundation of the hospitals that had been closed down, complained of 'the miserable people lying in the streete, offending every clene person passing by the way with their filthy and nasty savours [smells]' (quoted in Strype 1816, 424).

The immediate impact of Henry's dissolution of the monasteries was misery for many of those who had been cared for in religious buildings but also a 30-year gap in which little new building took place. The long-term effect was a fundamental shift in society's view of its obligation to disabled people. This started to become more a civic duty than a religious matter, although piety remained a fundamental part of the sense of obligation. Rich benefactors were no doubt still trying to save their souls, but were also intent on increasing their public esteem and flaunting the benefits that flowed from their wealth. New hospitals were built in London, and some of the old ones that had closed or suffered depredations under Henry's actions were refounded. These were now more public buildings, often ostentatious in appearance, their funding flowing from a mixture of parish collections, taxes, donations and endowments. Towards the end of the 16th century, after years of stagnation, new almshouses and hospital buildings started to spring up, now often less visibly linked to religious buildings, and more dispersed across villages and small towns (Bailey 1988, 90).

This process accelerated in the 17th century, culminating in the building of the two great hospitals for aged and disabled military veterans in London, the Chelsea Hospital for Soldiers and the Greenwich Hospital for Sailors.

There were also significant changes in the law. A series of Poor Law Acts enforced vicious punishments, including whipping and branding, for 'sturdy vagabonds', non-disabled beggars who were seen as idle and unemployed by choice. The so-called 'impotent poor', however, were seen differently. The 1531 Statute Concerning Punishment of Beggars and Vagabonds stated, 'The person naturally disabled, either in wit or member [mind or body] as idiot, lunatic, blind, lame etc., not able to work … all these … are to be provided for by the overseers of necessary relief and are to have allowances … according to … their maladies and needs.' This enshrined in law a distinction between the 'able' poor and the 'disabled' ('impotent') poor, the deserving and undeserving, a controversial distinction and debate which is still rehearsed today. These Poor Law developments also enshrined the principle that the state has some form of financial support obligation to people who have a disability.

Despite the proliferation of new buildings and the shift towards a sense of civic (and state) obligation towards disabled people, it remained the case that most people continued to live in their communities, with their families, surviving as best they could, just as they had in the medieval period. Life could be very hard indeed, but the idea of large-scale segregation or separation was barely considered.

The impotent poor – disability relief

Under the reign of Henry VIII from 1509 to 1547, the increasingly powerful Tudor state came to see itself as having a role in the regulation of poverty and the support of the most destitute, who included many disabled people. Three factors influenced this thinking. First, there was a change in public attitudes and new thinking about what government could do following the break from the Roman Catholic Church and the closure of monasteries in the 1530s, which until then had been the major institutional provider of care. Second, there was a new ambition and assertiveness within government about the scope of its activities, and a desire to control subjects and the lower classes. Third, harsh economic circumstances, including population pressure, accelerated poverty and distress and held out the potential for social unrest, mainly from a much-feared rootless population of unemployed 'vagabonds' (wandering beggars).

This brought about a raft of Poor Law legislation which sought to regulate the lives of the very poorest, particularly rootless beggars or vagabonds, but also to alleviate distress. It began, as we have seen, with Henry VIII's Statute Concerning Punishment of Beggars and Vagabonds of 1531. While this allowed wandering unemployed beggars to be whipped and returned to their parish of birth, it differentiated them from the 'impotent' poor (Fig 3.1). In the 16th century, this meant those unable to work through no fault of their own, usually because of disability, illness or old age. Under the statute the 'impotent' were allowed to have a license to beg in order to be able to avoid total destitution. This statute established the precedent of a sympathetic approach to those seen as not responsible for their own circumstances, the deserving poor, and the differentiation of those seen as unable to work because of a disability from those perceived as refusing to work by choice. It also earmarked disabled people as a legitimate subject for public assistance, who could be given relief support by their local parish.

In 1601 under Queen Elizabeth I, the last of the Tudor monarchs, the idea of a tax on local rate payers to be used for the support of the local poor was introduced for the first time, in the Statute for the Relief of the Poor. Every parish was allowed to secure funds to set the non-disabled poor to work and to relieve the impotent poor directly with cash. To do this they were given the legal power to levy a tax on all ratepayers.

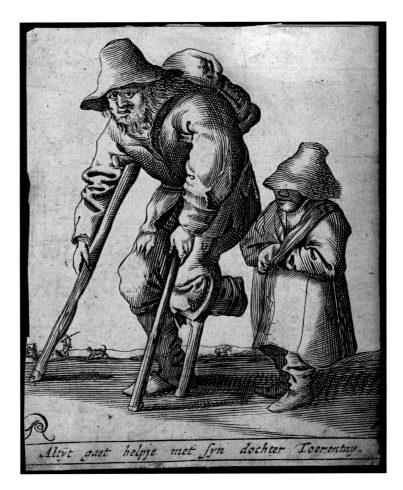

Fig 3.1
Impotent poor? A disabled
beggar accompanied by girl,
17th century.
[Engraving with etching by
P Quast. Wellcome Collection.
Public Domain Mark]

Altÿt gaet helpje met fyn dochter Toerentay.

This was Europe's first state-sanctioned system of poor relief financed by taxation, and remained so until the 19th century. Its main feature differentiating it from policy in the rest of Europe was that it funded mainly what was known as 'outdoor relief', which meant supporting people to live in their own homes in their communities with cash and in-kind relief, such as clothing or food. Only a small proportion was granted for 'indoor relief', which meant the parish paying for admission to workhouses or other institutions. This contrasted with the much more institutional model in much of Europe, such as the system of workhouses and almshouses in the Low Countries (broadly modern-day Holland and Belgium) or the huge hospital institutions for the destitute in France, such as the Salpêtrière (from 1656) and the Bicêtre (from 1642) in Paris. This community-based approach in Tudor England staved off any large-scale move towards institutionalisation, and meant that most disabled people, among them some of the most destitute, could continue to survive (although often barely) and function in the community.

The Elizabethan Poor Law therefore established four principles which would hold fast until the 19th century and have a profound effect on disabled people who were in poverty. Each parish was responsible for its own poor, the 'impotent' poor were to be maintained through poor relief, the non-disabled poor were to be set to work wherever possible, and a poor rate was to be levied on local middle-class and upper-class ratepayers to fund the operation of the Poor Law (Slack 1995, 1–50).

Poor Law records reveal how disabled people used these meagre parish grants and interventions to subsist. Interventions and support did not come automatically because a person had a disability. The expectation was always that the disabled person would live with their families and work if possible. Only when a person's disability and the fragility or absence of their family support network combined to place them at risk of total destitution would parish support occur. A small number of people we would recognise today as having learning disabilities – 'natural fools', 'innocents' or 'ideots' – were supported in this way, in cases where their families were struggling through ill health or extreme poverty. For example, in 1701 when Alice Stock, in the parish of St Botolph, Bishopsgate, London, became aged and lame, she received sixpence a fortnight to care for her 'foolish girle' Martha (Andrews 1996, 74).

If family care broke down or parents died, then 'keepers' or 'nurses' in the local community would be paid to care for people. The term 'nurses' is misleading to modern ears because these were not professionally qualified carers for the sick as we understand them today. They were, rather, local residents, male and female, who would take in a person needing care for a small remuneration from the parish. John Shusock of Wapping, London, was paid 2s 6d per week from 1649 to 1653 to 'keep' the 'innocent' (meaning learning disabled in modern terms) Thomas Walker, with extra payments for 'clothing and other necessaries' (Andrews 1996, 74, 83). Petitioners for aid from the Poor Law cited their own poverty, or deteriorating circumstances due to age or injury, when requesting support for a disabled relative. A woman in Northumberland described her husband as 'a simple man, and not in a capacity to manage their concerns'. She herself had become physically disabled through an accident, and they had become homeless, and were therefore forced to petition for relief. A footnote by the parish clerk in another case noted that 'the said James Twizell was born a foole which is the cause of his poverty' (Rushton 1996, 53–4).

Licencing of beggary for disabled people enabled them to be mobile across parish boundaries, searching for new and more lucrative sources of almsgiving, despite the difficulties created by their impairment. In the Stuart period, in the reign of Charles I (1625–49) a Nottinghamshire man claimed that he could walk 30 miles on a winter's day, despite being lame (Beier 1985, 70). Disease, disability, misfortune and accidents precipitated people into poverty, and then a precarious existence ensued, sustained by Poor Law donations and the proceeds of begging. As one historian has put it, in the 17th century 'disease and disaster generated licensed mendicants galore ... Parish records show endless processions of the deaf and dumb, blind, mad, shipwrecked, crippled, epileptics and fire victims' (Beier 1985, 112). There was an intimate connection between disability, either from birth or acquired by accident, and poverty, which situated disabled people among the most at-risk groups in early modern society.

Disabled people travelled to towns such as Bath and Buxton, where the waters were believed to have a rehabilitative effect, in search of cures. Travelling beggars and disabled pilgrims could be seen as a problem under the Poor Laws and greeted with hostility as they moved from parish to parish. Some were accused of impersonation of disability in order to attract sympathy or parish funds when begging, Often, parishes sought to evade financial responsibility for people, fearing that they would settle in the area and become dependent on poor relief, by moving them on or returning them to their place of origin. Treatment could be harsh. In 1622 an old man who was 'not able to go, stand or speak' was physically carried away by two men from Southwark in London to a neighbouring parish where he had previously lodged. Hertfordshire officials ordered the county closed to 'cripples, diseased and impotent persons' in 1625, because they were a 'great and unnecessary charge'.

The genuinely blind and disabled could be punished if they did not possess licences. An 'impotent woman' with a child was chastised for vagrancy in Oxfordshire in 1572, while in Windermere in 1635 a blind woman called Ellen Dixon was whipped, put in the stocks and then sent away. A man called William Clay, described as having 'no legs and is a vagrant and wicked liver', was incarcerated in Bridewell in 1640 and put to work making gloves. In 1652 Mary Wooles broke her back when she fell down stairs in London. She was sent to Bath after her legs gave way and her backbone started to protrude, but authorities returned her to London, from where she was sent to Wiltshire, and from there she was then sent back to London again (Beier 1985, 114–5).

The 16th and 17th centuries were therefore a period when the necessity of some form of state support, however minimal, for disabled people who were unable to work, was acknowledged and established in law. It was also a time when the combination of disability and poverty was lethal, leaving people to subsist as best they could, close to penury in the harshest of economic and social circumstances. Survival depended on the support of family and neighbours and, if this was unavailable, the kindness of strangers and Poor Law administrators.

Disability in the early modern city – the Norwich census

We gain an insight into the prevalence of disability and the lives led by disabled people in the crowded and unhealthy cities of Elizabethan England from the Norwich 'census of the poor' in 1570, 12 years after Elizabeth I had come to the throne. The census took place partly because of fears that the city would be overwhelmed by rampant begging among more than 2,000 paupers who lived in the town as forebodings of economic crisis developed. It was carried out as a precursor to reform of the administration of poor relief in the city.

The circumstances of 1,433 adults and 926 children, identified as the poorest in the city, were examined through a door-to-door survey. The census recorded information about sickness and disability as well as the family structure and the financial and living situation of each family (Fig 3.2).

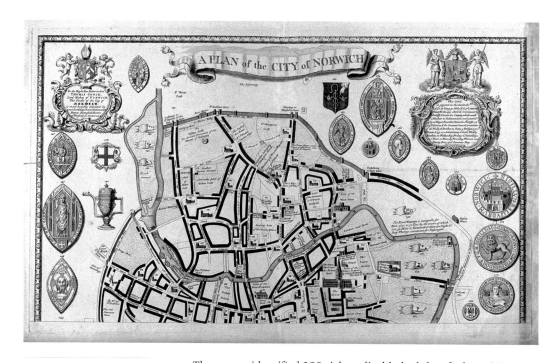

Fig 3.2

Norwich was an important early modern English city, with its share of urban poverty.

[Line engraving. Wellcome Collection. Public Domain Mark]

The survey identified 120 sick or disabled adults of whom 63 had some sort of long-term disability as opposed to an illness or disease. This group of disabled people comprised more women than men, 39 compared to 24. They divided into three main categories. By far the largest number, 44, had some sort of lameness, or 'crookedness', of legs, arms or their whole body. Fifteen had a sensory impairment: there were 10 blind and 5 deaf people. Four had missing limbs, with two lacking an arm or hand, and two without legs. We have no way of knowing how many of this group were born with their disabilities and how many acquired them through age, illness or accident. However, 28 people were aged 60 or over while only 9 were aged under 40. We might reasonably deduce from this that a significant number of people's disabilities were acquired with age. The imbalance between women and men overall is most marked in the over-60s, longevity offering some explanation why there are more disabled women than men (Pound 1971, 25–92).

The lives of the disabled respondents in the census were surprising. Almost all of the men and most of the women with disabilities were married to non-disabled people, and many had children. Their marriages were stable and long lasting (although two disabled women were identified as 'harlots', meaning prostitutes). Disabled people, though often poor, were an integral part of family life and work, closely networked in communities.

The lives of disabled and non-disabled respondents were strikingly similar. Just over half of the disabled people identified were married, while a further 13 were widowed. Nineteen were mentioned as having children, and only eight adults were living with their parents or with other families. Just 27 of the disabled group were unmarried at the time of the census. One woman had been left by her husband. There were significant age disparities between disabled people and their non-disabled spouses, which suggests that these might have been pragmatic remarriages based on 'a balance of abilities and disabilities with a view to common survival'. Notable among the disabled group are a 50-year-old blind man married to a 96-year-old woman and a 46-year-old lame man, an unemployed labourer, whose 80-year-old wife was still working as a spinner. Such cases suggest there may have been a pattern of mutually compensatory marriages, in which partners could help each other to manage their respective difficulties (Pelling 1998, 147–9).

Marriage rates for disabled people in the census were identical to the rest of the population, and the proportion of disabled women with children was identical to the numbers of non-disabled women with children (Pelling 1998, 18).

All of this suggests that disability represented no particular barrier to marriage for either men or women in comparison to the rest of the population. This was certainly the case for men, while for women marriage rates were lower but not significantly so. There was a small cohort of unmarried disabled women, most living with their parents. Marriages were invariably not between two disabled people, but between a disabled person and a non-disabled partner, although on occasions there were marriages between disabled people and sick or elderly partners. Disability was not seen as a particular barrier to having children. Levels of integration between disabled and non-disabled people were high, and expectations of marital relations and family life seemed to differ little between people who were disabled and people who were not. Disability was not seen as a reason for the non-disabled spouse to desert – there was only one marriage where this had occurred, a lower ratio than in the census as a whole.

Just under half of the disabled population identified in the census were, although poor, in work. The women were spinners or knitters, some of the 'lame' men were labourers. William Mordewe, a blind baker, was still working at the age of 70, aided by his young wife Helen. Some were unemployed but had a trade, including a hatter, cobblers and a carpenter. Only 12 people were specifically identified as unable to work because of their condition. The remainder were simply classified as 'not in work'. Just two people were beggars, both women, although it should be noted that vagrant disabled people would not have been picked up in this household survey. Employment rates were broadly in line with the main census population, although somewhat lower because of the 'not able' group.

The perception of disabled people as revealed in the census is that they were able, and expected, to work in most cases, and disability was generally not seen as a barrier to employment. Begging, on the grounds of helplessness or destitution, was a minority occupation. Being integrated to this extent can be viewed as a positive indication of the normality of disabled people's lives at this time and their natural acceptance in communities. It also indicates how having a disability was not an automatic route to getting some sort of parish support. Less than half of the disabled people in the census were in receipt of poor relief – most of them receiving between 1d and 3d a week, even though many of them were classed as 'veri pore' or 'miserable pore'.

Disability was no stranger to less populated rural areas. In Richard Gough's account of the parishioners of the Shropshire village of Myddle written at the beginning of the 18th century, disabled people are prominent in daily life. He refers to blind and deaf parishioners as well as a number of lame or 'crooked' people, including a young man with a steel plate fastened to correct his 'crypled' leg. While the disability of an individual is always referred to in Gough's account, the assessment and evaluation of their character was based on their individual personality – they were not defined, in his eyes, by their disability. Most of the disabled people referred to by Gough were married with families, and he is proud of the fact that only one disabled person, who was born blind, is dependent on parish relief (Gough 1988, 128, 145, 155).

Attitudes to disabled military veterans changed over this period, and there was a move towards providing greater support for those who had been wounded and left disabled by their participation in the numerous wars of the 16th century. Horrified at the sight of soldiers left to fend for themselves and die on the streets, senior captains agitated for hospitals, sick pay and pensions for those discharged with disabilities. This was gratitude for those who had sacrificed their bodies for the nation, but also an attempt to reduce the threat posed by vagrant soldiers on the streets. It was important that their disabilities be authenticated, however – a military certificate was needed for verification (Cruikshank 1968, 184–6). This was part of a wider suspicion of deception, particularly towards disabled beggars. Thomas Harman warned in 1566 of the so called 'Abraham [or Abram] Men', alleged fraudsters passing themselves off as destitute madmen, 'counterfeit cranks' dissembling the falling sickness (epilepsy) and the 'Dummerers' feigning inability to talk. He did, however, make a clear distinction between these roguish fakes and the genuine disabled beggar, whom he judged 'a cause of charity' (Harman 1972, 127).

Responding to mental illness

During his dissolution of religious orders, Henry VIII seized the Bethlem Hospital in London, England's only asylum for the mentally ill, whose medieval origins are described in Chapter 2. However, shortly before he died in 1547 he transferred its control to the Corporation of London, making it a civic, rather than religious, institution. In 1574, the city aldermen, struggling to keep it running, handed its management to the Bridewell, a hospital established for the management of the 'idle poor'. The Bethlem at this time could only admit a maximum of 40 people and was often only half full. The new governors had a strict admission policy, accepting only those people who were 'raving and furious and capable of cure, or if not yet are likely to do mischief to themselves or others' (Fig 3.3).

In 1619 Helkiah Crook became the first medically qualified 'keeper'. He was a controversial character who had accused the previous keeper of irregularities and who was constantly at odds with the Royal College of Physicians. His appointment indicated that, at an elite level, treatment of mental illness was starting to be seen as a medical skill rather than

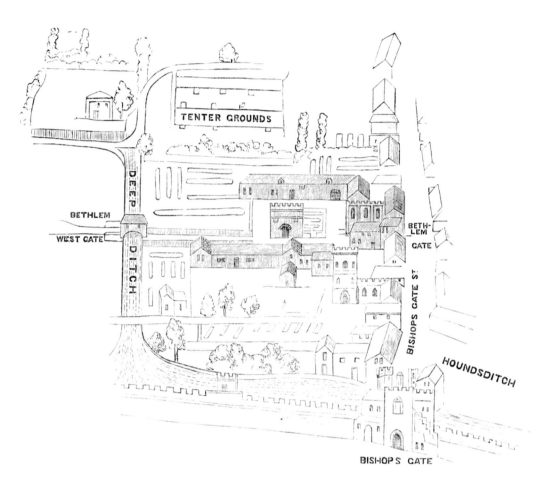

TENTER GROUNDS

BETHLEM

DEEP

WEST GATE

DITCH

BETH-
LEM

GATE

BISHOPS GATE ST.

HOUNDSDITCH

BISHOPS GATE

Fig 3.3
Plan of the first Bethlem
Hospital.
[From Daniel Hack Tuke,
*Chapters in the History of
the Insane in the British Isles*
(London, 1882)]

a matter for lay or religious people using traditional methods. Sadly, his medical qualification was all that distinguished him from previous keepers. A royal commission in 1632 found that he had been falsifying accounts and stealing donations while neglecting food and basic comforts for his patients. He was dismissed in 1633. His influence, however, was long lasting. The medicalisation of Bethlem's mental health care was now accepted as the norm. The hospital would, from this point, always be run by a medical officer with a team of medical staff (Andrews *et al* 1997, 55–144; Chambers 2009, 26–32).

It was only the handful of people with mental illness living in Bethlem and other small institutions who were receiving any sort of specialist institutional care in the 16th and early 17th centuries. In a population of five million, this meant that large numbers of mentally ill people remained in their communities, usually cared for by their family. Some were on the city streets and the country roads begging. Mentally ill beggars were nicknamed 'Tom o' Bedlams' (after the Bethlem hospital) (Fig 3.4). As with other disabilities, suspicion of whether a mentally ill person really was ill or was just feigning illness was widespread (Beier 1985, 115–16).

In the eyes of the law people deemed to be seriously mentally ill lacked the capacity to reason, and a Court of Wards would allocate responsibility for management of their affairs. On the whole they were not exploited through this system. King James I (1603–25) instructed the court that 'lunatics be freely committed to their best and nearest friends, that can receive no benefit by their death'. The care of the mentally ill was seen as a domestic matter.

Most people in Tudor England could not afford the services of a physician or surgeon, who mostly served only a tiny paying elite. There was, however, a vibrant 'medical marketplace' which was used by the poor and 'middling sorts', from which illness, including mental illness, could be treated. This offered up an eclectic array of practitioners – bone setters, wise women, cunning men, herbalists, astrologers – offering treatments. These could offer both natural and supernatural treatments, sometimes combined, for episodes of mental illness which, as in the medieval period, could be seen as caused by nature, devilish possession or even astronomical events. People had no difficulty holding these different explanations simultaneously.

Richard Napier was a clergyman, medical practitioner and astrologer who treated thousands of patients worried about their mental health between 1597 and 1634. People of all social classes, men and women,

Fig 3.4

Tom o' Bedlams – madness on the road as depicted in Shakespeare's *King Lear*.
[William Sharp]

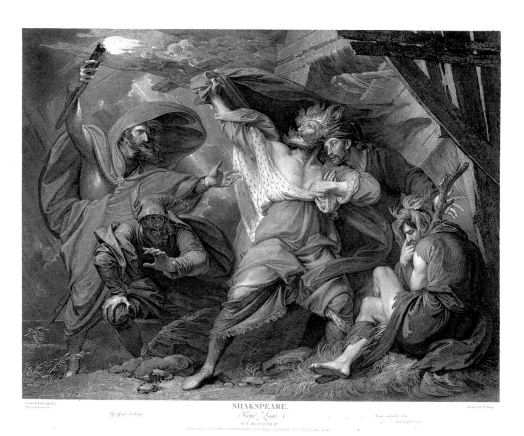

young and old, most of them not rich, flocked to his practice in the hamlet of Great Linford in Buckinghamshire. They included farmers, servants and labourers from his parish and the surrounding countryside as well as butchers, university dons, lawyers and, from the opposite ends of the social spectrum, the occasional beggar or member of the nobility (MacDonald 1981, 48–52).

Their symptoms included suicidal thoughts and self-harm, refusal to pray, inability to feel pious, sexual urges, visions, weeping, too much talk, and hatred of their spouse. Using religious, psychological, astrological and traditional healing remedies, Napier treated them all. Response to mental illness at this time, particularly in the hands of a relatively compassionate humanist such as Napier, could be as much about listening and humane intervention as incarceration in a building or ill treatment.

Napier recorded his consultations. Many were about the anxiety caused by economic misfortune, or the threat of it. One of his patients, John Scavington, was 'so crossed with debts that it broke his wits and senses'. Another, Robert Bell, who was also in debt, was 'mopish' and fearful, fearing 'that they will take away his goods and he will be undone'. Many of Napier's patients who needed treatment for mental disturbance had suffered some sort of terrifying or distressing experiences, with accidents and loss of loved ones common. Their lives were blighted by the threat of early death for themselves or their families through epidemics, consumption, parasites, dysentery, accidents, infections and botched childbirths. A patient of Napier called William Stoe was summarised by Napier as follows: 'Much grief from time to time. Had a wife long sick who died after much physic. Lost much cattle which died. Had the plague in his house; two children died [and he] himself had it … never well since.' The anxieties and depression caused by grief centred on the loss of close family members, child, spouse or parent, rather than on more distant relatives, friends or neighbours. Some were fatalistic, but others found their grief unendurable, lapsing into depression or even madness (MacDonald 1981, 67, 76–79).

Emotional turmoil could also cause mental distress. The young could be deeply affected by romantic disappointment. Napier wrote of a young woman called Jane Travell: 'Sayeth that nobody can tell the sorrow that she endureth … sometimes will sigh three hours until as sad as can [be] … Should have married one, and they were at words as if she would not have him. And then bidding him to marry elsewhere she fell into this passion. She noweth that she will never have him.' A young man called Thomas May threatened suicide if unable to marry the woman he loved: 'Grief taken for a wench he loves, he sayeth if he may not have her he will hang himself' (MacDonald 1981, 89).

Many women came to see Napier who were trapped, 17th-century convention and law giving them little freedom to escape, with brutal or philandering husbands. Mistress Podder told Napier she had been 'beaten blue around her eyes … mightily wronged and beaten by her husband that cannot brook her and calleth her a whore … her husband with his foot trampled on her chest, breast and belly.' The wife of Peter Ladimore, a curate, suffered mental distress because he 'loved another man's wife and kept her in the house … he drove away her own husband' (MacDonald 1981, 101).

Many of Napier's patients thought they were bewitched and were suffering mentally as a result. Witchcraft could be blamed for 'barrenness' (an inability to fall pregnant), stillbirths, illness and a host of other misfortunes, and was frequently attributed to the malevolence of neighbours arising from (often petty) disputes or arguments (MacDonald 1981, 108–11).

Napier applied a range of approaches and treatments to the mental anxieties and afflictions that his troubled patients brought to him. He employed divination to determine whether people were bewitched, conjuring up angels and using astrology and angelic magic to detect it and sometimes using prayers, charms, amulets and exorcism to cure. His many patients seeking consolation for their religious anxieties and fears (including their doubts of salvation) were recommended a sensible course of prayer, hope and religious exercises. Reflecting contemporary belief in the close interdependence of body and soul, there were also regimens of physical cure which closely resembled approaches to bodily ailments. Many of Napier's mentally disturbed patients were purged with emetics and laxatives and bled with leeches or by cupping (a form of suction). Drugs formed from plants, traditional recipes and inorganic compounds were given, many of them dating back to classical medicine. Tobacco was popular as a vomit (MacDonald 1981, 187–88, 220–22). It was clear from his notes that the simple act of unburdening their troubles to a sympathetic but dispassionate ear played a significant role in many people's road to recovery.

The heterodox approach adopted by Napier reflects the sheer breadth and range of symptoms that were affecting the people who came to him. There was something deeply pragmatic about his responses, and about the general attitudes that prevailed in 17th-century England, when faced with the unknowable workings of people's troubled minds. A potent mix of naturalistic, physical interventions with psychological, religious and supernatural responses offered at least some hope of easing the troubling complexities that undermined the mental stability of people facing economic, emotional and relational hardships.

New buildings for a new era

As we have seen, in 1485, at the beginning of the Tudor period, institutional care of disabled people was still largely in the hands of religious orders, in the 'spyttals' (hospitals) and almshouses run by orders of monks and nuns. While some remained well managed and honestly administered, there were growing concerns about neglect, abuse, building decay and corruption. 'I heare that the masters of your hospitals be so fat that the pore be kept leane and bare enough,' wrote one critic (Clay 1909, 224). After Henry's momentous divorce from Catherine of Aragon in 1533, and the consequent split from the Roman Catholic Church, the Church of England was established. Over the next 12 years the process of confiscation of the land, property and assets of the old Church, known as 'the dissolution', took place. Many hospitals, being religious institutions, were plundered and 'dissolved'.

The implications for disabled people whose care was undertaken and provided by religious orders were significant. Hospitals were targeted more by accident than design, caught up in the programme of hostility and plunder against anything which carried the imprint of the 'old religion'. Henry and his ministers appear not to have foreseen that this would lead to destitution for many sick and disabled people. Leading hospitals closed down, among them St Leonard's in York, St John Redcliffe in Bristol, Burton Lazars in Leicestershire and in London St Giles Holborn and St Bartholomew's. Bury St Edmunds lost 5 hospitals, including its leper house, York lost 13. The Maison Dieu (almshouse) in Dover became an ale house. As these institutions closed, those who lived in them were forced out. Many were left destitute. The king's attention was drawn to 'those miserable creatures which do now daylye dy in the streets for lack of their due porsion [portion]' (Clay 1909, 224).

There was a public reaction as the 'impotent poor' fought to survive on the streets. There was fear of the significant rise in 'sturdy vagabonds' but also concern for those seen as unable to fend for themselves: 'the pore impotent creatures [had] some relyfe of thyr scrapes, where as nowe they have nothinge. Then they had hospitals, and almshouses to be lodged in, but nowe they lye and starve in the stretes' (Clay 1909, 224).

At last Henry and his government were pressed into action by the petitions of citizens. In London, St Bartholomew's and St Thomas's hospitals were reformed and, with the Royal Bethlem asylum, passed to the control of the Corporation of London. Two new hospitals, Christ's for orphaned children and Bridewell for the 'correction' of 'habitual idlers', opened. These were now public hospitals, funded through donations, parish collections and taxes on companies. Their job was to implement public policy. Surviving hospitals and almshouses often passed to the control of civic authorities (Fig 3.5).

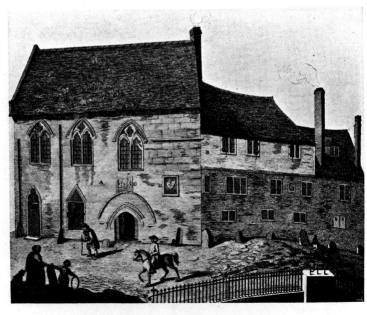

Fig 3.5
The Hospital of St Thomas, Canterbury, was among those that survived Henry VIII's dissolution.
[*The Medieval Hospitals of England* by Rotha Mary Clay: with a preface by the Lord Bishop of Bristol (1909)]

HOSPITAL OF ST. THOMAS, CANTERBURY

Some time after the upheaval of the dissolution, new almshouses and hospitals gradually began to be built again. John Port commissioned the Etwall Hospital in Derbyshire in 1557. Robert Dudley, Earl of Leicester, built a Maison Dieu in Warwick in 1571. In 1596 John Whitgift, Archbishop of Canterbury under Elizabeth I, founded the Hospital of the Holy Trinity in Croydon (Bailey 1988).

Coningsby hospital in Hereford was built in 1614 for 'eleven poore ould servitors that have been souldiers, mariners, or serving men'. Hospitals and almshouses were back, but they had become something different – secular institutions to look after those seen as not being able to look after themselves. Those who funded them aimed more to increase their public image than perform good work to ease their passage to heaven. If disabled people were seen as needing support, public rather than religious duty was now the driving factor.

From the small centres of religious care and refuge of the medieval period, some hospitals by the late 17th century had come to be seen as something far grander. They existed to be charitable and to protect public health – but also to express new ideas of public order and progress, particularly in the rapidly expanding capital of London. All of this had implications for disabled people in England, often seen as the objects of the charitable hospitals' care.

Attitudes to disabled soldiers changed over this period. Horrified at the sight of wounded men left to die on the streets, senior officers agitated for hospitals, sick pay and pensions for those discharged with disabilities. A small hospital for 'maimed soldiers' was founded in Berkshire in 1599, the precursor to much grander efforts in Chelsea, Greenwich and elsewhere in the later 17th century (Cruikshank 1968, 181–2). In Elizabeth's reign Acts were passed to provide pensions for soldiers and sailors who had 'lost their limbs or disabled their bodies'. The 'Chatham Chest', established in 1590 to pay pensions to disabled seamen, has been described as the world's first occupational health scheme (Cruikshank 1968).

Following the Great Fire of 1666, a London hospital rebuilding programme was launched to display the city's wealth and prestige. Surprisingly, this was led by the poor relation of the five London hospitals – the much discredited Royal Bethlehem, or Bethlem, London's 'asylum for the mad'. Though the old building was undamaged by the fire, the governors had concluded by 1674 that it was 'too weak and ruinous' and too small to meet demand. By 1676 a new building had been constructed in Moorfields, designed by the eminent scientist and architect Robert Hooke. Light and airy with landscaped gardens sweeping from the front entrance, it was designed to inspire awe and admiration and could house 120 people. One Londoner wrote 'so brave, so neat, so sweet it does appear / makes one half-mad to be a lodger there'.

The Bethlem's example inspired others. Charles II was keen to emulate Louis XIV's great Hôtel des Invalides military hospital in Paris and work began on Christopher Wren's Chelsea Hospital in 1682 (Fig 3.6). By 1691 (six years after Charles's death) this building for disabled and aged soldiers was complete. It would be followed by the Royal Hospital at Greenwich for disabled and aged navy veterans. These were grand buildings indeed, and the desire of the king to display to an admiring

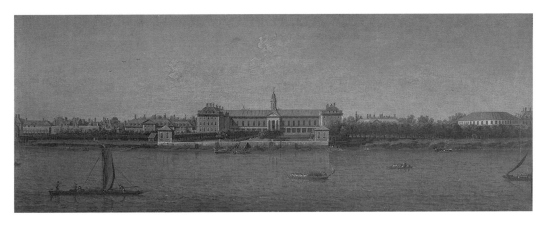

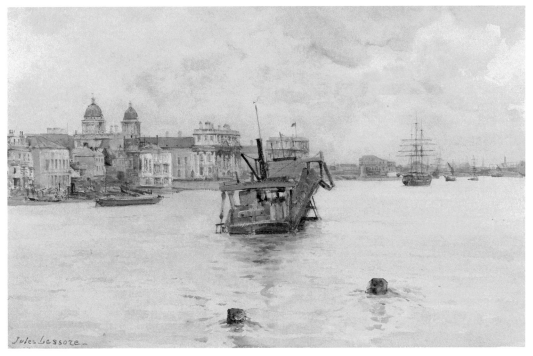

Fig 3.6
Chelsea Hospital for disabled
army veterans (1751, by an
anonymous artist).
[Tate]

Fig 3.7
Greenwich hospital for
disabled naval veterans (later
the Royal Naval College).
[Wikimedia Commons]

world his gratitude and esteem for those who had fought in his name,
and particularly those who had become disabled or infirm in doing so,
was clear. The Chelsea Hospital consisted of a single quadrangle which
opened onto a great terrace and causeway running down to the Thames,
beneath which were water gardens and orchards. Galleries, warmed from
large fireplaces, contained rows of individual cells (in the sense of private
rooms) for the inhabitants. The Great Hall contained large galleries
where groups of veterans ate at tables for each 'mess'. Great staircases
connected the different levels of the building. Greenwich, begun in 1696
but not finally completed till 1764, was equally grand with its colonnades,
courtyards, galleries and sweeping vistas down to the river Thames
(Stevenson 2000, 53–61, 71–84) (Fig 3.7).

It had become the mark of a great commercial trading nation to display its commitment and obligation to those who had sacrificed their bodies in defending its cause, but also to show off its opulence, success and formidable military might to any who might dare to doubt or challenge it.

The lives of disabled people

When Thomas Speller married Sara Earle in St Botolph, Aldgate, London, in 1618 it was an unusual occasion. Thomas, a blacksmith, was a 'dumbe person' and indicated his willingness to marry Sara by making 'the best signes he could, to show that he was willing to be maried'. Permission had been given for the ceremony to go ahead after the Lord Chief Justice had agreed that a marriage could be solemnised without the vows being actually spoken by one of the parties. Thomas Speller and Sara Earle, therefore, give us the first known English wedding conducted in sign language (Forbes 1971, 29).

Twenty-five years later, in 1643, another deaf man made his mark on history. As the English Civil War (1642–51) reached Lichfield in Staffordshire, John Dyott, aged 37 and nicknamed 'dumb Dyott', was part of the Royalist forces defending the town against an assault by Oliver Cromwell's parliamentary forces. From the battlements of the central cathedral spire a bullet fired by Dyott killed the commanding officer of the parliamentary army, Lord Brooke. Dyott was led back into the town to a hero's reception from the people of Lichfield. After the civil war he married a young 'deaf and dumb' woman called Katherine and they had four daughters and a son. This was one of the earliest ever recorded marriages between two born-deaf people (Jackson and Lee 2001, 55).

Much attention has been paid in historical writing to the presence of so-called 'fools' in royal courts, employed to entertain the monarch and courtiers, the humour usually at their own expense because of their foolery. There has been much speculation over whether such people were 'natural' or 'artificial' fools, in other words whether they were born with some form of disability or whether they were just 'playing the fool' in their role as court entertainer. In reality, both sorts of fool were employed in courts. However, we should remember that the importance of such people has been somewhat overstated in the history of disability because of their prominence and visibility, and their presence in court archive material. The existence of a small number of natural fools among the royal elite is, though, a matter of some fascination, and gives some insight into prevailing attitudes.

One of the best-known court fools who was almost certainly a 'natural' is William Somer, a fool to Henry VIII from around 1535. Although well paid, well fed and well clothed in return for his work in Henry's court, Will Somer did not lead the same life as other courtiers. In 1551, some years after Henry's death, a payment of 40 shillings was made to William Seyton, 'whom his Majesty hath appointed to keep William Somer'. Somer needed a 'keeper', a person who would look after and care for him, and was clearly understood not to be able to care for himself. This strongly suggests that he was a 'natural fool'. Despite this, Somer was highly regarded and wore fine clothes. When he was first recruited to the court he was fitted out with

> a dublette of wurstede, lined with canvas and cotton … a coote and a cappe of grene clothe, fringed with red crule [wool embroidery] and lined with fryse … a dublette of fustian, lined with cotton and canvas … a coote of grene clothe. With a hoode to the same. Fringed with white cruel lined with fryse and boherham [buckram].

Somer was famous for his witty and blunt speaking to Henry. He is reputed once to have said: 'As please your Grace you have so many frauditers, so many conveyers and so many deceivers to get up your money, that they get all to themselves.' The words should have been 'auditors, surveyors and receivers' and he was telling his monarch through this joke that he was being defrauded and exploited by those around him. Few in the Tudor court would have dared speak such an uncomfortable truth to Henry, but Somer's humourous, and yet truthful, banter was much loved by the king. As a fool, he had licence to speak the truth in ways that others could not. This was in the tradition of the 'holy innocent', who lacks guile, pretention or malice and therefore cannot but help tell truth to power. This characterisation is a long-standing stereotype about the learning-disabled person where their simplicity and lack of understanding about the malicious guile of other people causes them to speak simple truths (Southworth 2003, 91–103).

Henry's previous fool Sexton, known by the nickname Patch (meaning 'fool'), was also considered a 'natural' who needed help and support in his life. He had been 'given' to Henry VIII, along with Hampton Court Palace, by Cardinal Thomas Wolsey, the Lord Chancellor, who was desperately trying to win back Henry's favour as allegations of treason were made against him. It was recorded that it took six tall yeomen to transport the clearly distressed Sexton to the court. A succession of 'keepers' or carers were paid to look after him and given funds for his needs, such as food, laundry, shoes and 'posset ale'. Clothing was provided for him, rather than purchased by him with his own money. However, like other 'natural fools' in Henry's court, Sexton did not wear the harlequin's motley and cap with bells familiar to us from images of court jesters of this period. He wore high-quality cloth and silk doublets and coats, the clothes of a favoured retainer (Southworth 2003, 85–90).

Another prominent 'natural fool' of the 16th century was 'Jane the fool', who appears to have been the 'woman fool' successively of Anne Boleyn, Henry's second queen; Princess Mary, his daughter; and, from 1546, Katherine Parr, his sixth and last queen. Court records show that Jane was expensively clothed at the court's expense and there were eight payments at 4d a time for 'shaving of Jane [the] fool's head' (Southworth 2003, 130–6).

Paintings from this time show the prominent positions occupied by 'natural fools' in the royal family. A 1545 painting shows Henry VIII with his 'ideal family' – his long-dead favourite wife Jane Seymour, his son Edward and his daughters Mary and Elizabeth. Will Somer and Jane the fool appear on either side of the painting, flanking the family (Fig 3.8).

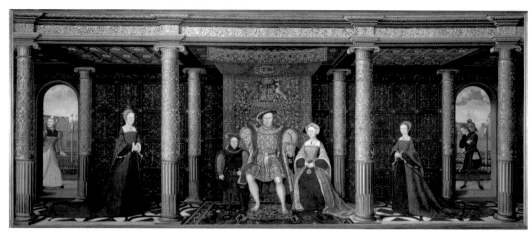

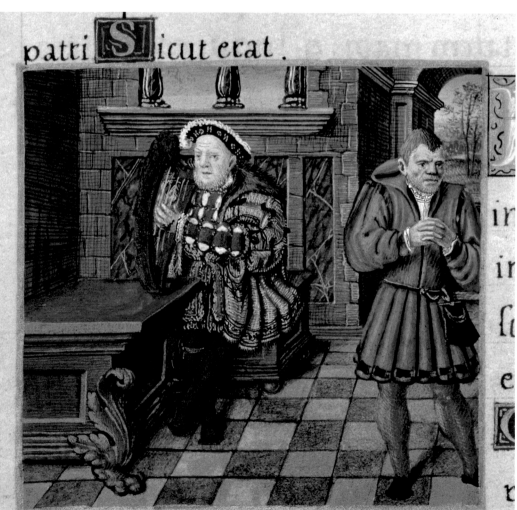

Another intimate family portrait shows Somer between Henry and his three children, and an illustration from 1540 in Henry VIII's personal psalter shows the king and Will Somer acting out psalm 52 of the Bible – 'the fool says in his heart there is no God'. Somer is wearing the green cloth hooded coat specified in the wardrobe account (Fig 3.9).

These glimpses of 'natural fools' in the Tudor court show people seen as naturally 'foolish' occupying valued and significant roles in the lives of the Tudor elite. Their perceived lack of guile, their directness and their humour were recognised as assets and woven into the fabric of court life. Seen as closer to the truth than other people, they occupied a unique and surprising position.

Fig 3.8
Henry's ideal family – Henry VIII with family including Will Somer (right) and Jane the fool (left).
[Royal Collection]

Conclusion

The 16th and 17th centuries saw significant changes in the lives of disabled people in England. While religious belief and piety remained almost universal, there was a shift away from the religious model of care, carried out by monks and nuns in religious buildings, that had characterised the medieval period. This process was hastened and made explicit by Henry VIII's dissolution of the monasteries in the 1530s, which destroyed many places of care and refuge for disabled people who made use of them, initially causing great hardship. However, this ushered in, from the end of the 16th century, more secularised and geographically diffuse forms of building-based care in almshouses and hospitals. New hospital buildings, such as the Greenwich and Chelsea military veteran hospitals in London, the new home for the Bethlem hospital in London's Moorfields and the profusion of almshouses across the country were often more a testament to the wealth and power of their founders, and the state, than to God. Royal backing and funding for the elegant and lavish veterans' hospitals was also a statement about England's commercial and military might.

However, the continuity with the medieval period was that most disabled people went nowhere near an institution of care, but lived as everyone else did. They could be found everywhere. They might be licensed beggars at the roadside, sustained in part by Poor Law funding for the 'impotent', or well looked after and remunerated retainers of the royal court. They might be an active participant in England's civil war or making a living well into old age in the poorest quarter of Norwich. Wherever they were, and whatever they were doing, they were present, and noticed, embedded in their families and communities, accepted and participating in the struggles of daily life.

Discussion: The place of special communities

Fig 3.9
Henry VIII with his 'fool' Will Somer.
[British Library]

As we have seen, Henry VIII's dissolution of the monasteries saw many disabled people having to leave the religious houses where they were cared for, leading to calls for new institutions to replace them. But there has always been a debate about whether people should live separate or integrated lives. Do separate communities and separate schools offer something or are they just another contributory factor to the isolation and marginalisation of disabled people?

One of the watchwords of 21st-century disability rights activism is inclusion, the right of people to be equal citizens of the same communities and societies as non-disabled people, with the same entitlements and opportunities. This reflects the exclusion of disabled people over time, which has taken many forms. People have been excluded from work (and therefore economic independence), from buildings and from sites of social interaction because of both access and acceptance problems, and from being able to enjoy the same leisure and social opportunities as non-disabled people. In some instances people with some forms of disability have been excluded from political life, denied the right to vote or to participate in democratic processes. In its most extreme form, exclusion places a barrier between the person labelled disabled and the rest of society, confining them to locked and isolated institutions such as asylums, effectively cut off from the world.

Today the debate about separation or inclusion goes on. Do some disabled children need separate special schools or should all children be part of mainstream education? Do disabled people need to use separate specially adapted buildings, such as day centres, or should all buildings be fully accessible and integrated so that there is no need for separation? Is it right that disabled people have the opportunity to work in sheltered work settings, or should it be the norm that everyone works in mainstream, open employment?

The special village community

The 20th century has seen a very distinctive example of separate living, where disabled people have lived in specially created, self-sustaining communities, apart from the rest of society – the special village. These are sometimes known as 'intentional communities' – meaning that in principle people only live in them if they choose to do so and have expressed a considered wish to live there. They see themselves as distinct from institutions, such as asylums, because they are structured on family and community life. Inhabitants live simple lifestyles, in a self-enclosed, largely self-supporting community. They belong to the tradition of the commune, which has existed in English society since the radical religious sects such as the Diggers of the mid-17th century. Communes flourished again briefly during the 'hippy revolution' of the 1960s and 1970s. Internationally, the Kibbutz movement in Israel and the Anabaptist communities of North America (Amish, Moravian and Hutterite), which originated in 17th-century Germany, exemplify the separate, self-sustaining community.

An early example of an English village community of disabled people is Enham Alamein, near Andover in Hampshire (Fig 3.10). Built in 1918 as the Enham Village Centre, this was the first specially created village for the care and support of disabled servicemen returning from the First World War. It was aimed at men unable to return to their former trades because of their disabling injuries and focused on supporting them to regain independence and earn a living wage. Crucially, servicemen

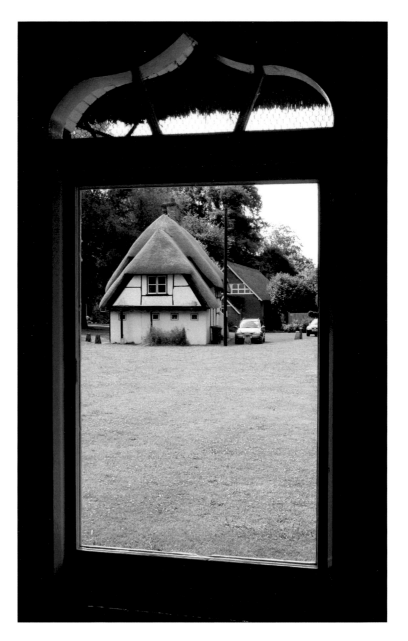

Fig 3.10
A view of Enham Alamein,
established as a village
community for disabled war
veterans.
[Mike Cattell]

were able to settle in the cluster of houses with their families, creating a genuine community. Those who lived in the village were known as 'settlers'. In its rural setting, the village contained craft workshops, a poultry farm and facilities for book and shoe repairs, furniture making and upholstery. With its own woodworking factory and market garden, it aimed for as high a level of economic independence as possible. Fulfilling industrial orders for the Second World War effort, including the manufacture of gliders, brought Enham to its highest level of self-sustainability.

After the Second World War, Enham, with a new generation of disabled war veterans to house, was boosted by a financial gift expressing the 'gratitude of the Egyptian people' in commemoration of the battle of El Alamein in 1942 between British and German and Italian forces. Renamed Enham Alamein, the village saw new purpose-built cottages and flats added in the 1940s and 1950s. New industries, such as candle making, were introduced. Enham Alamein survives today as a community providing housing and work training for people with learning and physical disabilities.

Camphill communities

The origin of the Camphill communities is extraordinary. The first Camphill School was founded by a group of German and Austrian Jewish refugees from Nazism. Led by the inspirational paediatrician Karl König, a Christian convert, they wanted to create a new form of 'healing environment' for the education and upbringing of children with special needs. Following the teachings of the social reformer and educational philosopher Rudolf Steiner, they rejected the fashionable idea of the time that some children were ineducable. They wanted to create a community where children with disabilities and (unpaid) staff would live together and share their lives to foster mutual help and understanding. They believed that there was 'in each human being a hidden and eternal soul' that had to be reached.

They began with their first community in Aberdeen in 1940, where Scottish children with learning disabilities were educated by, and lived with, mainly Jewish refugee educators. The daily language of the school in its early years was German. The movement flourished and the first English community was built at Botton Village in North Yorkshire in 1956. Today there are 22 communities in England, for both children and adults, and many more around the world (Fig 3.11). Influenced by the Moravian Christian communities of North America, 'villagers' (also known as 'Camphillers') live as 'co-workers' in non-hierarchical communities. Family-sized groups live together in small houses. Mostly in rural settings, the communities produce high-quality hand-crafted goods and foods, as well as sustaining themselves with their own produce. Some villages have their own gift shops and cafes. Their cooperative businesses include agriculture, horticulture, cheese making, pottery and woodcraft. Simplicity, naturalness, tranquillity and respect for the 'natural rhythms' of life are key. Villagers come together in a central village hall to celebrate Christian festivals, changes in the seasons and the rhythms of the farming year. Buildings are simple, with as many natural materials as possible used. Camphill is now an international movement, operating in 23 countries.

Towards the end of his life, Karl König recalled what it was that brought together this unlikely alliance of exiled European Jewish intellectuals and British children with learning disabilities. Why did they end up together in their own special community, outside mainstream society? 'The handicapped children, at that time, were in a similar position to ours. They were refugees from a society which did not want to accept them as part of their community. We were political, these children social, refugees' (König 1960, 15).

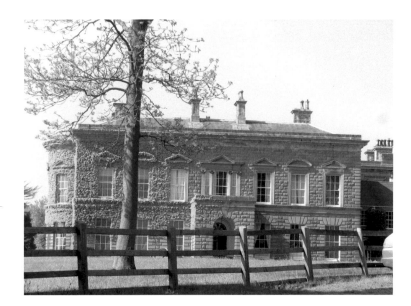

Fig 3.11
The main house in the
Camphill Community,
Oaklands Park,
Gloucestershire.
[Quichot (Edwin Klein)]

König's words are important. We tend to think of 'community' as a
necessarily good thing. But as König knew only too well, and as many
disabled people have always known, communities can turn on their
minority members, or those they designate as not belonging, in life-
threatening ways. Sometimes a separate community such as Camphill
Aberdeen, with its unlikely alliance of Jewish intellectuals and learning-
disabled children, is created because the wider community represents an
existential threat.

Conclusion

The debate about the intentional community outside mainstream society
can be a complex one, more complex than it might first appear in an age
which sees itself as 'inclusive' and opposed to any form of separation.
Tom Shakespeare has captured the two sides of the argument well. Such
communities, he writes,

> seem to provide safe and sheltered environments where people …
> are supported within family structures, engage in work and can have
> freedom to live normally. Yet this is achieved by creating a rather
> segregated and unusual rural village situation, in which very motivated
> non-disabled people live with a high proportion of people who need
> support.
>
> (Shakespeare 2014, 207)

He notes that such ways of connecting can appear patronising, but
adds that 'such relationships can develop into important and mutually
satisfying connections' in which the 'benefits outweigh any anxieties
about charity or paternalism which disability rights activists have
sometimes expressed' (ibid).

4 Age of elegance? The 18th century, 1714–1800

Introduction and summary

In the 18th century important shifts took place in the understanding of disability. English social attitudes continued the move to a more secular and less religiously dominated outlook that had begun in the Tudor period. While the idea that disability and madness had some sort of God-given or other supernatural cause did not disappear, and religious piety remained the overwhelming norm, punitive notions of sinfulness and possession diminished in importance and there were new explanations, including secular ideas.

Madness came to be seen more as a loss of reason than some sort of possession of the soul and so it became accepted that with the right treatment, reason could be restored. Disability could be seen more as a misfortune than a mark of sin or holiness. It was also seen as part of God's overall plan: if a person had a disability this was God's will and therefore the disabled person, like the poor, the rich, the less intelligent and the genius, occupied their allotted place in the great chain of being. Everybody had their place in the hierarchy and, so long as they accepted it, then they belonged. This essentially conservative doctrine was a brake on social mobility and the alleviation of poverty, but its rigid structure contained a form of acceptance. If God had bestowed forms of disability on some people, then those people belonged just as much as those to whom God had allotted better fortune – things were what they were.

This prevailing outlook, known as 'optimism', which accepted whatever God gave as the way of the world, was satirised by the French philosopher Voltaire in his novel *Candide* (1759). His anti-hero Dr Pangloss, who continually states that 'all is for the best in the best of all worlds', whatever the evidence to the contrary before his eyes, is an unshakable proponent of the theory of optimism. Voltaire demonstrated its absurdity. Nevertheless, the creed of optimism saw people with any sort of disability as functioning within society (provided they knew their place) rather than outsiders who should be excluded.

Disability was therefore worthy of charity, a part of the Christian and civic duty to ease the suffering of the poor. Disabled people generally saw themselves as part of their communities, who would marry, work and support themselves if they could, and were entitled to the help of the better off if that proved impossible. For the most part support for disabled people was seen not as the duty of the state but as the charitable duty of the individual. The parish might step in with poor relief but, as we have seen, for this to happen disability was not sufficient in itself: a person had to be destitute as well. As a disabled person you belonged to society, but you were subject to its harsh and brutal vicissitudes like everyone else, probably more so (Fig 4.1).

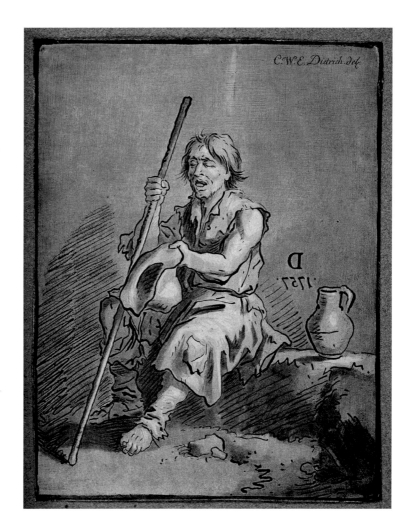

Fig 4.1
Disability, being God-given,
was seen as worthy of charity
in the 18th century.
[Coloured Mezzotint by C W
E Dietrich, 1757. Wellcome
Collection. Public Domain
Mark]

Important social and cultural changes were taking place. London, a booming, rapidly expanding global city, the largest in Europe, wanted to show off its ever-growing wealth and power. The massive building programme which had taken place after the Great Fire of 1666 continued as the city expanded throughout the 18th century to become the largest capital in the Western world by far. Hospital building took place across the country as England (and Britain from 1707 after the act of union brought England and Scotland together) grew into an important commercial and military power. New naval hospitals were built to house aged, sick and disabled sailors and veterans. Towards the end of the century a voluntary asylum movement sprang up, led in part by the Christian Quaker sect, based on a belief that both disabled and mentally ill people could flourish in healthy, clean institutional settings. Alongside all this emerged that unique English institution, the private madhouse, situated in non-purpose-built houses, and mostly catering for the mentally distressed of 'the better sort'.

A belief in civic order and progress spawned many new institutions. The charity school movement for education of poor children was followed at the end of the century by the first specialist schools for 'deaf and dumb' and blind children. This growth in institutional specialist provision for differing forms of disability reflected wider trends. An Enlightenment belief in the primacy of scientific medicine as a rational response to bodily imperfection challenged the hands-off precepts of the school of optimism. Everything, it was thought, including disability and disease, could be solved through reason and scientific exploration. Human progress would flourish if only the right environments could be created for the march towards perfection. The notion of perfectibility, however, was an ominous mode of thought for hitherto assimilated disabled people, and accompanying it were the first stirrings of the age of the institution as the century drew to a close.

Despite all this, in daily life most people with any sort of disability continued to live in society at all levels. They ranged from disabled beggars using ingeniously created technologies fashioned from scraps of wood to assist their navigation of the teeming city streets, to distinguished and socially esteemed deaf portrait artists.

Physical impairment

As in previous centuries, disability could often mean destitution, as most people's livelihoods depended on the ability to do hard physical work. The preponderance of disabled beggars on the London streets was remarkable – urban pedestrians were warned in 1716 to beware of crossing Lincoln's Inn at night, an overnight haunt of beggars, for fear they would be knocked down with their crutches. But if the disabled poor were seen as a hazard by some non-disabled persons, the packed streets of England's cities, particularly London, were far more hazardous to negotiate for disabled people. They could also be, with their frenetic coach and cart traffic, an actual cause of death for them. A former prize fighter called William Metcalf, who was lame as a result of a 'great sore on his leg', died in London 1731 after his 'stick or crutch' was caught in the wheel of a dray cart, causing him to fall under the wagon. In 1765, another lame man, William Smalley, was crushed to death crossing the Haymarket when he was unable to get out of the way of a cart (Hitchcock 2004, 11; Turner 2012, 141–2).

The halt, the lame, the crippled (as they were called) were everywhere, as were the unusual methods they used to make themselves mobile. The better off were able to purchase specialist medical appliances and assistive technology, such as trusses (for ruptures), crutches, artificial legs, arms and hands, along with dubious medicinal spirits and balsams which, their vendors claimed, would enable the immobile to get up and walk (Turner 2012, 52–3).

The poor had to resort to fashioning their own ingenious technologies from wood (Fig 4.2). Roughly hewn crutches and sticks, cleverly adapted to the person's particular range of disabilities, enabled poor disabled people to negotiate the streets as best they could. Their technologies were such a familiar sight that they passed into daily slang usage. 'Billies in bowls' were beggars who lacked their lower limbs, who sat in hollowed out wooden tubs, propelling themselves with two small wooden blocks

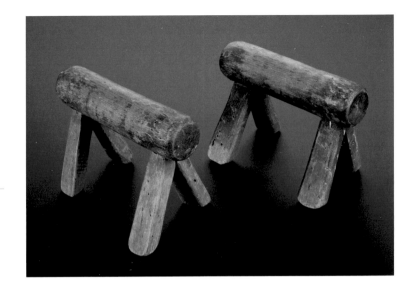

Fig 4.2
Pair of 18th-century wooden
hand crutches.
[Science Museum, London.
Attribution 4.0 International
(CC BY 4.0)]

held as crutches. The most famous of these was 'Philip in a Tub', an actual character from London's streets in the 1740s who is depicted in William Hogarth's *Industry and Idleness* series, selling ballads outside a wedding. He is notable for his immensely muscular arms, honed by his daily life of hauling himself around the streets (Figs 4.3 and 4.4). There were also 'go-carts [or karts]', roughly constructed wheeled boxes in which the disabled person would sit and be pulled either by a dog or a helper. It was from these that our modern term go-kart (or go-cart) is derived. 'Sledge beggars' sat on curved wooden bucket seats and either propelled themselves or were pulled through the streets by a dog or a person (Hitchcock 2004, 110).

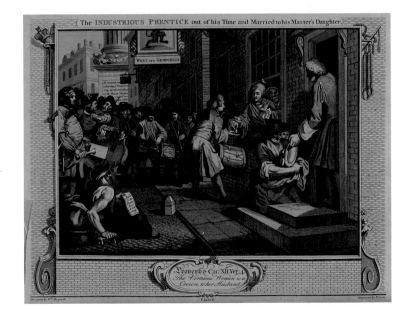

Fig 4.3
'Philip in a Tub' sells ballad
sheets outside the wedding of
the industrious apprentice in
Hogarth's morality tale.
[Engraving by Thomas Cook
after William Hogarth.
Wellcome Collection. Public
Domain Mark]

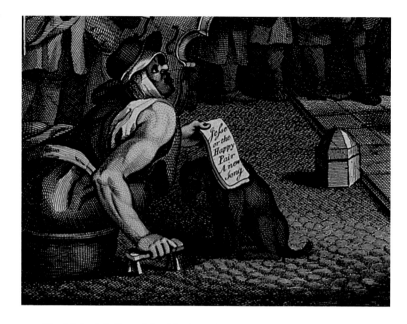

The high visibility of disabled people in everyday life meant that there were a small number of people, like Philip in a Tub, who might be called 'disabled celebrities'. Crowds gathered to watch a street artist, described as 'a poor cripple, known about town for his ingenious writing on the pavement'. There were those who made a good living from the display of their disability and the fascination of the public, including high society, with their 'remarkable' bodies. Matthew Buchinger, 'the little man of Nuremburg', came to England in the early part of the century (Fig 4.5). He was said to be 'but 29 inches high' and lacked 'Hands, Feet and Thighs'. He exhibited himself at the court of George II and other London venues and was admired for his talents in playing 'various Sorts of Music to Admiration, as the Hautboy, Strange Flute in Consort with the Bagpipe, Dulcimer and Trumpet'. He was also admired for his abilities in writing and drawing true-to-life pictures, and for having married four times, siring 11 children. He earned well from his performances. This public interest could be seen as voyeurism and inappropriate fascination with a 'deformed' body, yet it is also true that Buchinger was admired for his remarkable abilities and skills, and he was certainly the agent of his own fortune (Turner 2012, 84–5, 95–6).

The medieval idea of the divine miracle cure had largely disappeared, treated with scepticism and even mocked in the English press, seen as a relic of Catholic superstition. Levels of anti-Catholic hostility were high in England for most of the 18th century, fuelled by the threat of Jacobite rebellion (seeking the restoration of the Catholic Stuart monarchy) and deep anti-French feelings. The *Daily Journal* in 1736 poked fun at Rome, which it said was 'all in a surprise' at the miraculous cure of a nun, 'a perfect cripple', as a result of looking at a picture of the deceased wife of James Stuart, the Jacobite claimant to the English throne. The idea of disability as a mark of sin also waned, although it still carried some cultural import. Medical practitioners, both formal and informal, took

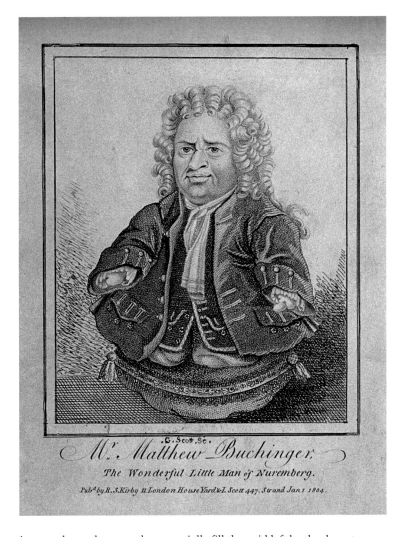

M.ͬ Matthew Buchinger.

The Wonderful Little Man of Nuremberg.

Pub.ᵈ by R. S. Kirby 11 London House Yard & I. Scott 447. Strand Jan 1 1804.

it upon themselves to at least partially fill the void left by the departure of the miraculous cure. They advertised 'cures' for lameness such as electricity, spa waters, bonesetters, powders and patent medicines. A famous bonesetter, Sally Mapp, held aloft the crutches of those whose bones she had allegedly set straight as 'trophies of honour' (Turner 2012, 41, 50–51).

Impairment was a matter of degree and there was no overarching category of 'disabled people' which marked them out as unable to work and in need of support. In fact, people were expected to work for as long as possible and to do whatever was within their ability. Even the loss of a limb was not an automatic obstacle to employment. Those who became disabled would often be forced to move from skilled to unskilled work, and thus into greater poverty, but the expectation was that they would continue to work. At an Old Bailey trial in 1793, Arthur Driver, a witness, described how he worked as a labourer from 3.00 am to 9.00 am. He had previously been a seaman, but was wounded and became lame. In

1776 William Young, previously a pin maker, was 'disabled by the loss of one eye' and forced to earn a precarious living as a 'tickets porter', eventually having to seek charity to survive (Turner 2012, 129). Low-paid, precarious casual work was the norm for many disabled people, and included mending shoes, sweeping crossings for pedestrians or selling goods on the street such as birds, oranges, vegetables and old rags (Turner 2012, 129–30).

As had been the case since the medieval period, care and support if needed came from the family and neighbourhood, rather than in any sort of institutional setting. Although low levels of Poor Law funds were available for the chronically destitute, the expectation was that parents should support their children, husbands their wives (and vice versa), and adults support their aged parents. Thus disability could bring about poverty and hardship in an entire family. William Trudger told Poor Law overseers in Essex that his family had fallen into poverty because of his daughter's regular fits, which meant that her mother had to look after her rather than work. Such cases indicate the devotion of families to their disabled family members and their willingness to suffer hardship and invest resources to look after them. This contrasts markedly with the often-held belief of some historians and commentators that disabled people were marginalised and ostracised, even disposed of, in this period.

Disabled people had their own thoughts about how they might lead their lives, and were not passive bystanders as others decided their fate. They could be skilled at couching their appeals to Poor Law administrators and other authorities in such a way as to secure the maximum benefits possible, and were not averse to threatening that they could become even more of a burden if not properly recompensed. Disabled petitioners often claimed that their pensions were too small for them to subsist, or their earnings too low to survive without assistance, and would warn overseers that without help they would be 'coming to your poor house'. Petitioners would constantly stress that despite the limitations imposed on them by lameness or other forms of disability, they wished to be socially and economically independent and had no wish to be considered a burden on the parish. They did not see themselves as victims, nor did they have any desire to be seen as such (Turner 2012, 139–40).

'Idiocy'

People categorised as idiots or imbeciles during this period, broadly the terms for those we would call people with learning disabilities today, occupied an integrated position in 18th-century society, even if acknowledged and understood as different by their families and neighbours. The few specialist institutions of the time, such as the Bethlem hospital, Guy's and the correctional Bridewells in fact actively sought to exclude so-called idiots. This was because it was recognised that such people did not have some sort of curable or treatable disease, but were simply a type of person who had in some areas of functioning different levels of mental faculty to most others. For them to be assigned to a place of cure or treatment therefore made no sense, and the medical profession continued to show barely any interest in this group.

Court records from the Old Bailey, London's criminal court, testify to the integrated lives that people led in their communities. So-called idiots appeared before judges and juries, sometimes as defendants, usually accused of minor offences, but sufficient to entail the death penalty if found guilty under the harsh 18th-century penal system, known as the 'Bloody Code'. They also appeared as witnesses and victims, and their family and friends often spoke about them in court.

Leniency was often shown by judges and juries even when it was clear that an 'idiot' defendant had clearly committed a crime, as this trial from 1710 demonstrates:

> Mary Bradshaw, alias Seymour, of St Giles without Cripplegate was indicted for feloniously stealing 2 stuff gowns, value 20s, a Stuff Petticoat 3s with other things, the Goods of Elizabeth Morgan. A cloth petticoat 5s a Stuff Petticoat 3s, 3 Dowlace Smocks 15s, the Goods of Anne Downing. The Fact was plainly prov'd upon the Prisoner, but sufficient Proof being given in Court that she was an Idiot, the Jury acquitted her.
>
> (OBP 1710, quoted in Jarrett 2020, 42)

Mary Bradshaw was thus spared the hanging that her offence warranted, judge and jury making a judgement either that she was to be pitied or, more likely, that she was harmless and could be taken care of by her family or neighbourhood to ensure that she did not reoffend. Such verdicts were common. In 1748 Robert Left, on trial for stealing a brass weight, was acquitted by the jury, who 'said they thought he was an idiot'. As late as 1804 'Charles Viton was indicted for feloniously stealing … one pair of breeches, value 12s … It appearing to the Court that the prisoner was an ideot, or lunatic, and subject to fits, he was acquitted' (Jarrett 2020, 42).

The trials reveal that many named as idiots in court held down jobs and lived within networks of family and friends. In 1780 a young learning-disabled man, Thomas Baggot, who collected animal skins for making leather at Newgate market in the City of London, was saved from the hangman's noose when his employer, workmates and family all gave (contradictory) evidence that he had not participated in the anti-Catholic Gordon riots, despite an eyewitness testifying that he had. Witnesses would attest to the good character of their so-called idiot friends, neighbours and workmates. They would invariably describe a character who was intellectually weak but morally strong and respectable: 'a very honest, but a very silly ignorant fellow'; 'I never heard anything amiss of him, but took him to be a little soft (or foolish)'; and 'I always was of opinion that he was soft, but with respect to his honesty, I never heard a bad character of him in my life', were typical examples (quoted in Jarrett 2020, 44).

Close relatives would plead on behalf of their family members, emphasising their foolishness and vulnerability but also their harmlessness and the love of their family for them. The mother of John Longmore, on trial for assault in 1732, stated: 'He is a harmless, half-witted, foolish lad.' One witness explained that his brother, on trial for theft, had been affected in his behaviour by damage that had been caused

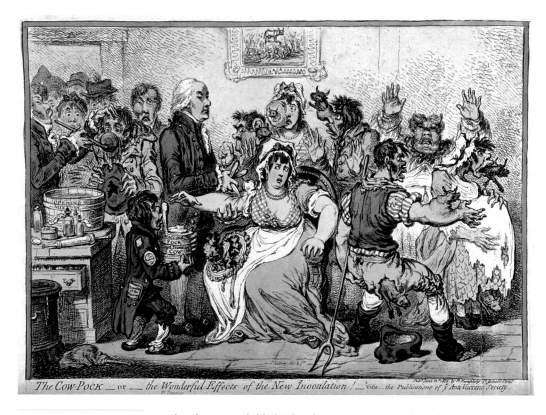

The COW-POCK _ or _ the Wonderful Effects of the New Inoculation ! _ Vide. the Publications of ỹ Anti Vaccine Society.

Fig 4.6

'Idiots' lived and worked in their communities in the 18th century, as in this depiction of Edward Jenner's servant (bottom left) carrying the cow pock (smallpox) vaccine. [Coloured etching by H Gillray, 1802. Wellcome Collection. Attribution 4.0 International (CC BY 4.0)]

when he was a child: 'his head was torn to pieces by a dog when he was two or three years of age'. Relatives would also seek compassion and urge sympathy, promising that the defendant would stay out of trouble in the future if the jury would show mercy. The father of 'foolish' epileptic Elizabeth Camell, also accused of theft, appealed to the judge and jury saying: 'she is all the children I have out of fifteen. God bless you use her as well as you can. If she is released I'll take care to send her far enough from London if she has got into ill company' (quoted in Jarrett 2020, 44).

Some people named as idiots in Old Bailey trials were married. John Thomas was described by his father-in-law as 'a simple lad, little better than an idiot'. Sarah Holloway's husband accompanied her after her arrest and described her as 'silly … and when anybody has given her a farthing, she has stood laughing for half an hour; they used to call her Foolish Nan'.

Many also worked, and workmates and employers would testify on their behalf. Women worked largely in menial jobs, often as servants, chars or washerwomen (Fig 4.6). The 'half-natural, very silly creature' Mary Radford carried out charring tasks for rich households. Some laboured in the marginal economy, such as Ann Terry who worked 'closing upper leathers for shoes'. She was part of an organised group of pauper women in London known as 'translators', who took old shoes that had been begged or found and gave them new soles. She was described in court as 'a very silly foolish girl, not capable of taking care of herself'. Robert Miller survived by running errands for gentlemen. He was described as 'much troubled with fits, and half an ideot' (quoted in Jarrett 2020, 84).

People worked in more stable occupations too. The labourer mentioned above whose head was 'torn to pieces' by a dog when he was two, whose name was Peter Cunniford, had worked in a building company for 12 years and was viewed by workmates as 'a hardworking, honest fellow'. Although many males described as idiots were employed as unskilled labourers or servants of some sort, a small number were in skilled occupations, such as bricklaying, carpentry and paper hanging. Some were even involved in running small businesses, although usually with some help. John Bullock kept a public house in Essex, but he was a 'silly innocent sort of a fellow … the management of the business lay altogether up on the wife' (Jarrett 2020, 84–5).

These intriguing glimpses into the lives of people classed as idiots in the 18th century suggest that they were people who lived at the heart of their communities, loved by their families and accepted by their neighbours and workmates. They lived and worked in a variety of settings. Being an idiot did not in itself define a person. They could be seen as contributing workers with rounded personalities. The situation should not be over romanticised – other trials provide evidence of cruelty and ridicule, with witnesses testifying: 'I have seen 'em black his face. And carry him about in a basket, and then throw him out into a kennel [gutter]'; 'he is a poor silly fellow, laughed and jeered at by the rest'; 'people used to push him about and ill-use him' (quoted in Jarrett 2020, 85). If people were perceived as vulnerable or undesirable, they could easily be ostracised or attacked by sections of the community. However, in all the instances of violence and bullying cited, there was a response from other community members who stood up in defence of the person concerned. The idiot's place in the community, however tough it may have been at times, was an integrated one.

Madhouses and 'madness'

The beginning of a creeping institutionalisation of madness is apparent in this period. The Bethlem Hospital sat in its proud and elegant new surroundings at Moorfields, built towards the end of the 17th century, with capacity for 120 patients. But behind the elegant façade lay a disturbing reality (Fig 4.7). Over the 18th century, Bedlam was run by the medical dynasty of the Monro family. Dr James Munro was succeeded by his son John, who was succeeded in turn by his son Thomas, in turn followed by his son Edward. The acquisitive Monros would become a byword for the corruption, neglect and, often, ill treatment that had always characterised the institution. William Hogarth famously depicted Bedlam as a hellish den of unregulated madness and suffering, poorly treated lunatics in his *Rake's Progress* series of 1732–34 (Fig 4.8).

This century of corrupt neglect culminated in an inspection by reformers in 1814 which revealed shocking conditions and abuses. In the female galleries patients were chained by an arm to the walls, naked apart from a blanket gown. In the men's wing, they were chained by both an arm and a leg. Many were incontinent, and straitjackets, leg locks and

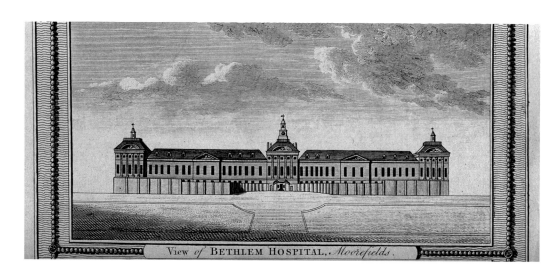

View of BETHLEM HOSPITAL, Moorfields.

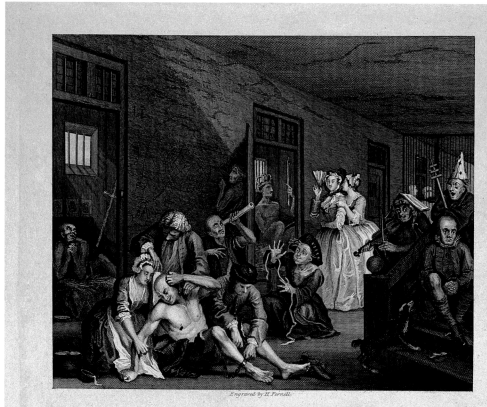

Engraved by H.Fernell.

THE RAKE'S PROGRESS.

PLATE 8

SCENE IN BEDLAM.

From the Original Picture by Hogarth.

other forms of restraint were in use. An American sailor called James Norris was discovered who had been locked up for 14 years and who, after trying to defend himself against ill treatment by his keeper, was confined by an iron contraption built around his neck and head which prevented all movement. He had been confined in that way for 12 years. The eminent John Haslam, resident apothecary at Bethlem, and Thomas Monro the physician, were both dismissed at the subsequent enquiry, where each tried to blame the other for Bethlem's woes. But their fates were immaterial – Bethlem, or Bedlam, had been woven into the English imagination as a place of horror, where madness and cruelty collided to create unendurable misery (Scull *et al* 1996; Porter 2002, 97).

Despite the enormity of its reputation, Bethlem remained insignificant in terms of the number of the so-called mad who passed through its doors. It was an exception, as a hospital-type institutional setting for people with mental illness, but because of its reputation, location and the disturbing stories that it constantly generated, it impacted heavily on the public consciousness.

Quietly in evidence, and much less noticeable than the garish cascade of horror stories that gushed from Bethlem, was a unique feature of English society in the 18th century: the private madhouse. Madness was coming to be seen as the loss of reason rather than something with a divine cause or remedy. It could be restored through what eventually became known as 'moral treatment': gentle discipline, order and well-intentioned manipulation. And what better place to do this than in the orderly, well-managed institution of a small private madhouse, with its family atmosphere and controlled environment?

Rarely purpose-built, by the end of the century there were around 45 of these officially licensed private dwellings adapted for the accommodation of 'the mad' around the country. They catered largely for better-off residents, particularly the smaller houses which charged the highest fees and accommodated only five or six people. There were a few larger houses which housed some 'pauper lunatics' paid for by the parish. In such establishments, living areas for paupers and private patients were strictly segregated and of widely differing quality (Parry-Jones 1972, 29–127).

From the 1790s, at the very select Ticehurst House in Sussex, patients could bring their own servants, some lodging in their own dwelling in the grounds of the large house (Fig 4.9). A pack of beagles was kept so that gentleman patients could enjoy the hunt. Work was very important for the restoration of reason. At the Greatford Hall madhouse in Lincolnshire run by Dr Frederick Willis, famous for treating George III, 'the unprepared traveller … was astonished to find almost all the surrounding ploughmen, gardeners, threshers, thatchers and other labourers attired in black coats, black silk breeches and stockings, and the head of each *bien poudrée, frisée et araignée* [well powdered, curled and styled]. These were the doctor's patients.' Many homes advertised their extensive gardens, or pleasure grounds, which were often walled to prevent wandering. The better houses might have a bowling green, a small library and indoor games like bagatelle (Porter 1992, 287; Parry-Jones 1972, 183–4).

Behind the high ideals and optimism, however, there was disquiet about treatment in these private institutions and standards varied widely.

Fig 4.7
The new Bethlem Hospital at Moorfields was soon as mired in scandal as its predecessor. [Engraving, 1775. Wellcome Collection. Public Domain Mark]

Fig 4.8
Hogarth's famous depiction of madness in the Bethlem Hospital in his *Rake's Progress* series (1732–33). [Engraving by H Fernell after W Hogarth, 1735. Wellcome Collection. Public Domain Mark]

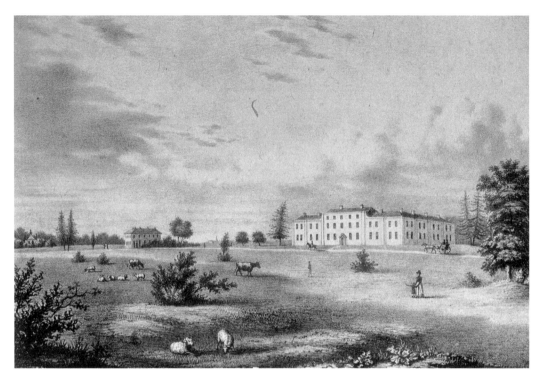

Fig 4.9
At Ticehurst House patients
could bring their own
servants.
[Wikimedia Commons]

In 1763 *The Gentleman's Magazine* condemned the 'many unlawful arbitrary and cruel acts' which went on in madhouses. At Lainston House near Winchester, private patients resided in the mansion, but paupers, some of them incontinent, were kept in converted stables and outbuildings. The home was eventually closed for mistreatment of its paupers, who had been left chained in cold and filthy conditions.

The proprietors, known as mad doctors, were a varied group and not necessarily medically qualified. They had little social or professional status and included clergymen, quack doctors and family dynasties. Medical qualification bore little relation to quality of care. This depended more on the charitable instincts and motives of the proprietor, like those who ran the more reputable institutions such as Brislington House in Somerset and Laverstock House near Salisbury. From 1774 the Regulation of Madhouses Act introduced a licensing system, following public concern that some non-lunatics were being unlawfully detained at the whim of their spouses or families. With the growth of state-managed county asylums in the 19th century, the private madhouse declined, although several survived in some form through to the 20th century.

Despite the presence of a small number of institutions, most people experiencing mental illness sought remedies and support within family and community settings. If they had the financial wherewithal, they would see a practicing mad doctor for a private consultation. Wealthier individuals sometimes arranged for their servants or other employees to have such consultations. John Monro (1715–91), who was the physician at Bethlem for 40 years, had a busy private practice in London as well as supervising the institution, and one of his books of case notes has survived. It gives an intriguing insight into the mental health concerns of worried individuals and their families who came to him.

Many illnesses were strongly influenced by religious concerns. In 1766 Monro saw Miss Jeffries of Welbeck Street, an unmarried woman aged 46 who he described as 'very low, imagines herself to have been very wicked, & her Distemper to have brought on by her own imprudence & has attempted, & talks very deliberately of putting an end to her life, her brother was either an Idiot or a Lunatic & died under confinement' (Andrews and Scull 2003, 5–13, C1–C124). Another patient blamed his sinful masturbatory habits when younger for his depressive mood: 'Mr _____ came to me to relate his case which was of the low-spirited proceeding, as he said, from having been guilty of Onanism to a great degree when young. He was once before in this way.'

Some had visions of devils and other foreboding apparitions: 'M Walker, a distiller in Shoreditch whom I called upon this morning told me the devil left him this morning about 4 o' clock that he had been with him 7 years, was brown and of a size between a mouse & a rat. He informed me that there … the world was near it's [sic] end.' A person's own sense of sinfulness often drove their unwelcome thoughts: 'Miss Greaves the 3rd or 4th relapse a family misfortune, imagines nothing she does is right, & that she is thus plagued for the sins she has been [?], has bad thoughts. Sleeps but little and is afraid of seeing knives, bits of string & c.' Others were tipped over the edge by misfortune or disturbing experiences. When Monro went to see Mr Sergison, a coachmaker in Kensington who had been 'disordered' for about a fortnight, his family attributed his mental ill health to his recent experience as a juror at the Old Bailey (Andrews and Scull 2003).

There is rarely any record in his notes of how Monro treated these complaints; his role was perhaps reassurance to families and a listening ear for those who were unwell. There are references to people going to the country for restorative air and quiet, or sometimes taking prescribed powders. Notes were sometimes added to say that within a short time some people recovered: 'she got well and I took my leave of her June 6'. Despite his role at the Bethlem Hospital, Monro rarely seemed to discuss confinement for his private charges – even for a mad doctor, family was the prevailing place for care to take place.

In a reaction against the depredations of Bethlem and the dubious reputation and slow decline of the private madhouse, a lively charitable movement began which sought to pursue the social aims of supporting the sick and disabled poor rather than create buildings of grandeur. In 1712 the charitable Bethel Hospital for lunatics was built in Committee Street (later Bethel Street), Norwich. In 1721 Guy's Hospital in London opened its doors, built for incurably sick and chronic lunatics.

St Luke's, a rival and near neighbour to Bethlem, was a charitable asylum for pauper lunatics built in London's Old Street. It kept to the tradition of grandeur with a magnificent classical frontage but adopted a very different approach to the care of the mentally ill. Run by the eccentric physician William Battie, it advocated (but did not always achieve) a system of non-restraint, occupation, fresh air and good food, and rejected the Bethlem-type regime.

Other voluntary hospitals sprang up. Small-scale asylums each housing around 100 people were built in Manchester (1766), Newcastle

Fig 4.10
William Tuke, founder of the
York Retreat.
[Wellcome Collection. Public
Domain Mark]

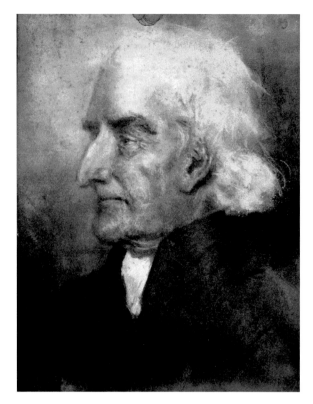

Fig 4.11
The York Retreat.
[Wellcome Collection]

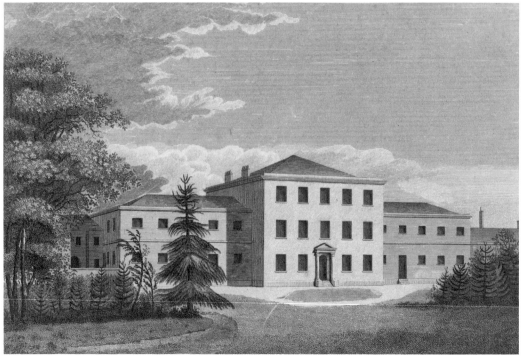

(1767), York (1777) and Liverpool (1792). Voluntary did not always mean good, however, and York became notorious for corruption and abuse. In 1796, the Quaker community, led by William Tuke, chose to establish their own asylum, the York Retreat in Bootham. 'Medical' treatment was replaced by 'moral' means – kindness, reason and humanity in a family atmosphere, with no restraint (Fig 4.10).

The Retreat became famous around the world. In England the foundations were in place for the era of the asylum and the institution for those deemed mad (Fig 4.11).

Blindness and deafness

Here is an 18th-century joke about a blind woman.

> One Easter Monday, an arch-rogue meeting a *blind* woman who was crying *Pudding and Pies*, taking her by the arm said Come along with me Dame, I am going to Moorfields, where this Holliday time, you may chance to meet with a good Custom. Thank 'e kindly sir, says she. Whereupon he conducted her to Cripplegate church, and placed her in the middle isle. Now says he, you are in Moorfields: which she, believing to be true, immediately called out, *Hot puddings and pies! Come, their* [*sic*] *all hot!* And so on, which caused the whole congregation to burst out in a loud laughter, and the clerk came and told her she was in a church: *you are a lying son of a whore* says she. Which so enraged the Clerk, that he dragged her out of the church: she cursing and damning him all the while, nor would she believe him 'till she heard the organs play.
>
> (Anon, nd)

The joke is very shocking to our 21st-century ears. A practical joke is played on a blind woman (a poor street-seller at that), so that she ends up crying out her wares in the middle of a church service on an Easter Monday, thinking that she is on the streets of Moorfields. The congregation cannot contain their laughter. Yet if the joke is examined more closely it can tell a different story. Once again, it indicates to us that in this period disabled people, including those who were blind, were expected to make a living, and were working in the heart of their communities. The woman, old blind and poor as she is, is no victim. 'You are a lying son of a whore' she bellows at the clerk of the church. She gives as good as she gets. Most of all, the joke – unpleasant as it may seem to us now – is testament to the embeddedness of blind people in 18th-century society. They were not hidden away, or afraid to come out onto the streets. In fact, in real life outside the world of the joke, deaf people were sometimes allowed to sit near the front of the congregation in church, a position normally only given to worshippers of higher status (Turner 2012, 88).

The portrait of 'The Curds and Whey Seller' from the mid-18th century by an anonymous British artist shows the reality of blindness on the streets (Fig 4.12). The saintly looking blind woman holds out her hand for payment from the mischievous young chimney sweeps who have bought her wares, but they tease her by not paying the correct

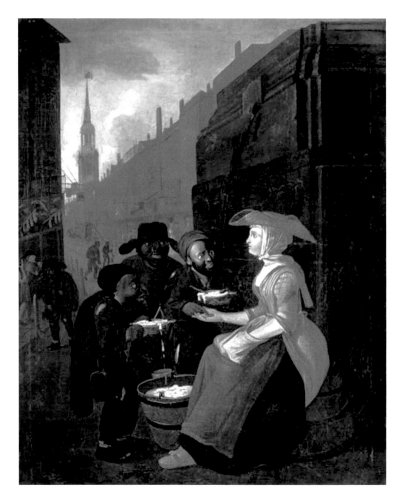

Fig 4.12
The blind curds and whey
seller of Cheapside.
[Wikimedia Commons]

money. To be occupying her place on the streets selling curds and whey she needed to be part of a network of selling and distribution, supplied with her goods each morning, making her way to her pitch, known to the passers-by, engaged in transactions of exchange, and returning home each evening.

The Foundling Hospital in Bloomsbury, London, and other institutions taught blind children to play a musical instrument, and a blind violinist, cellist or other instrumentalist playing for money on the streets was a common daily sight (Hitchcock 2004, 115). Blindness enabled an appeal for charity and compassion which often elevated the blind person in the hierarchy of disability, whatever the casual cruelty of some jokes suggested. To be blind, suggested a letter to *The Gentleman's Magazine* in 1807, was not 'half so pitiable' as being deaf, because 'the pleasures of conversation and the charms of music can much alleviate their want of sight'.

Restoration of sight for some became a possibility as medical advances made 'couching', the removal of cataracts, possible and more frequently practiced. Oculists advertised these successes as miraculous victories over blindness, in their efforts to attract new customers seeking the same: 'A few days since, Master Smith, son of Captain Alexander Smith of Lombard Street by Mr Taylor, Oculist of Hatton Garden, after being deemed incurable' (quoted in Mounsey 2019, 43).

However, as one historian of blindness has noted, blind people on the whole did not expect to be cured, and saw themselves as disabled, but they also did not see themselves as separate or belonging to some marginalised group (Mounsey 2019, 276). Each simply had their own life experience, and dealt with the difficulties blindness brought to them as best they could.

Deafness was equally common, and the experiences of deaf people equally varied. At the lower end of the social scale, the deaf poor found themselves doubly disadvantaged, and in desperation some turned to whatever way they could find to survive. The prostitute Elizabeth 'Betty' Steel (1764–95) was, in 1787, the first deaf person transported to Australia – she had assaulted and robbed her (deaf) client in a pub in notorious Black Boy Alley, Holborn, London (Jackson and Lee 2001, 172–3).

At the other end of the social scale, in the golden age of portrait painting at the end of the 18th century three remarkable deaf miniaturists, Richard Crosse (1742–1810), Sampson Towgood Roch (1759–1847) and Charles Shirreff (1750–1831), flourished as high-society artists in London and Bath. Crosse became court painter in enamel to George III. The artist Joshua Reynolds (1723–92), who became deafened at the age of 26 after a fall from a horse, was the first president of the Royal Academy. He believed that his deafness sharpened his vision and increased his insight into his sitters. This was the idea of the 'compensatory faculty' popular at the time, which claimed that if you were deficient in one part of your body it would be made up for by increased faculty in another part. It is believed that his sister Frances, who kept house for him, acted as his interpreter using gestures and mouthing words. Disability also reached further into the royal court at St James through Duncan Campbell (1680–1730), who was presented to George I in 1720. Campbell was a 'deaf and dumb' man who worked as a 'professional predictor', or clairvoyant, communicating with his clients by writing, gestures or finger spelling. 'All his visitors come to him full of expectations', reported *The Tatler* sceptically, 'and pay his own rate for the interpretations they put on his shrugs and nods' (Jackson and Lee 2001, 37–8, 48, 155, 156, 167).

In education, although a thriving charity schools movement providing education for the children of the poor took off in the first half of the 18th century, it did not include disabled children. Those from better-off families could enjoy private tutoring or take their chance in the small number of mainstream schools, but the disabled children of the poor were unlikely to receive an education. This began to change towards the end of the century, as the first deaf and blind academies were established.

In Gloucestershire, Thomas Arrowsmith (1771–*c* 1830) (Fig 4.13), who was born deaf, was taken aged four or five by his mother to the local village school where she demanded that he be educated. Despite the misgivings of the teacher, he was admitted and did well. He then became

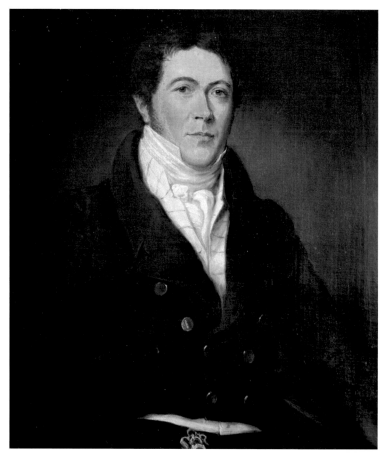

Fig 4.13
Thomas Arrowsmith, a
distinguished graduate of the
Braidwood Academy for the
deaf and dumb.
[Wikimedia Commons]

a pupil in England's first special educational provision for the deaf –
Braidwood's Academy for the Deaf and Dumb in Grove House, Hackney,
on the eastern edge of London. Thomas went on to become a well-known
painter, studying and exhibiting at the Royal Academy, the first of a
number of distinguished graduates of the Braidwood Academy (Jackson
and Lee 2001, 5–6).

Thomas Braidwood (1715–1806) set up the academy in London in
1783, having run a successful school in Edinburgh since 1760. He used a
form of sign language known as the combined system (later known as the
Braidwoodian system), which was the forerunner of British Sign Language.
He had dreamed of setting up a public school for poor deaf children.
However, it was one of his pupils, John Creasy (c 1774–1855), who inspired
and persuaded his local reverend to raise money to build the London Asylum
for the Deaf and Dumb in Bermondsey in 1792. This was the first ever public
school for the deaf in England. A former pupil, William Hunter (1785–
1861), later became Britain's first deaf teacher of the deaf. This had, said the
head teacher, 'the happiest effect' of a deaf teacher communicating with deaf
pupils in their own manner (Jackson and Lee 2001, 47, 103).

Meanwhile, a young man from Liverpool, Edward Rushton (1756–
1814), survived a sinking on a slaver ship heading for Dominica. Outraged

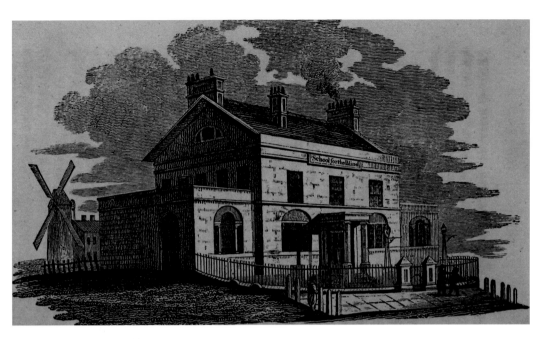

Fig 4.14
Edward Rushton's personal
experience of ophthalmia led
him to found the Liverpool
School of Industry for the
Indigent Blind.
[Wikimedia Commons]

at the brutal treatment of the slaves on the ship, he was charged with
mutiny after remonstrating with the captain. He tried to assist the slaves
with food and water. Many of them had caught the highly contagious
ophthalmia and he contracted the disease himself, losing the sight in one
eye and becoming virtually blind in the other. On his return he became a
poet, anti-slavery campaigner, newspaper editor and general supporter
of radical causes. However, his most lasting legacy was the Liverpool
School of Industry for the Indigent Blind, in London Road, Liverpool,
which opened in 1791 (Fig 4.14). It was the first specialist school for the
blind in the country, second in the world only to Paris. Pupils were taught
music, weaving, basket making, spinning and other trades to equip them
for economic survival and independence after school. The school survives
today (in a new location) as the Liverpool Royal School for the Blind.
Inspired by Rushton, blind schools were built in Bristol (1793), London
(1799) and Norwich (1805).

Through innovators such as John Creasy, William Hunter and Edward
Rushton, the principle that young deaf and blind people had the right to an
education, and the ability to pursue it, was established. It was at this point
that the idea of specialist education for disabled children and young people
began to take off, an idea which has caused controversy and debate ever
since.

Hospitals, almshouses and workhouses

The construction of the Greenwich Hospital for sailors at the end
of the 17th century was the prelude to a century of naval hospital
building for wounded, disabled and infirm sailors and veterans. The
Haslar Hospital in Gosport, Hampshire, opened in 1762, followed

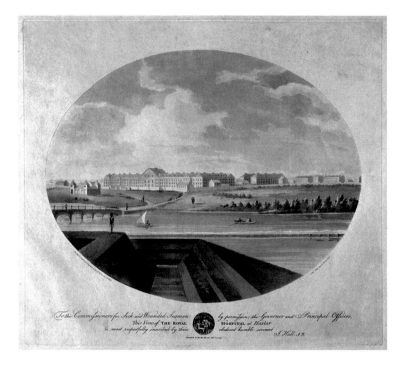

Fig 4.15
The Royal Hospital, Haslar,
in 1799.
[Coloured aquatint by J Wells,
1799, after J Hall. Wellcome
Collection. Public Domain
Mark]

by Plymouth (1762), Deal (1795) and Great Yarmouth (1811). This
spate of building represented a move to a more permanent setting,
and the opportunity for longer occupation by veterans, as opposed to
the more temporary use of hospital ships that had preceded the land-
based hospitals. They reflected both the enormous size and strategic
national importance of the Georgian Navy and were suitably grand in
both conception and design. Haslar had 114 wards, most of them with
19 or 20 beds. There were two enormous wards of 52 beds each. The
hospitals were characterised by large galleries, courtyards, gardens and
sweeping views – Haslar sat in 30 acres (Fig 4.15). These institutions
were regarded as models of good practice and care unrivalled in Europe.
Their primary aim was to treat illnesses and diseases, such as scurvy,
and to make sailors fit for service again. However, they were also an
important recognition of a growing sense of obligation to those who had
been wounded and disabled in the service of their country. They were
instrumental in creating a category of heroic disabled veterans to whom
the nation felt indebted, a viewpoint which endures today (Rodger
1986, 109–12; Stevenson 2000, 172–94).

Almshouse building for the infirm, disabled and elderly recovered
slowly from the post-dissolution dip, and the shift from religious to
secular donors continued. They found themselves in competition with
poorhouses, which local parishes were now enabled, and encouraged, to
build using Poor Law taxes. With the state, often via the parish, assuming
greater (if somewhat reluctant) responsibility for the 'impotent' and
destitute poor, private charitable donations for almshouses remained
fairly stagnant. Nevertheless, endowments persisted and for the lucky few
the perils of disability and infirmity in old age were eased by the chance

to pass the last years of their lives in the relatively comfortable and secure surroundings of an almshouse. New buildings arose in Avon, Yorkshire, Shropshire, Leicestershire and Lancashire, suggesting a northward spread away from the dominant south-east. The end of the 18th century saw a distinct decline in almshouse building, caused in part by growing industrialisation and the expansion of cities, and also the economic hardships and preoccupations brought about by the Napoleonic Wars (Bailey 1988, 141–60).

From the 1720s onwards there was a significant expansion in parish provision of poorhouses, also known as workhouses. Such was the expansion that by 1776 in London there were 86 workhouses, from virtually none at the beginning of the century. These were frequently used as places of temporary refuge or for other purposes by the disabled poor. Eighteenth-century workhouses were of a very different nature to the punitive prison-like institutions that would arise in the 19th century, which will be discussed in the next chapter. Although there was a structured regimen that meant permission was needed to gain leave, and occupants could sometimes be set to work, there was little coercive restraint and people were generally encouraged to go out to work, beg or seek other accommodation. For the poor, and particularly disabled people in need, they offered somewhere to stay for a few nights or more, food and clothing, and were also closely aligned with the parish network. Sometimes these short stays would develop into permanent residence for those too incapacitated to live or work elsewhere. They ranged in size from St George's Hanover Square in London, which could accommodate several hundred people, to small workhouses taking just half a dozen people. The larger houses were often used for parish meetings and almost all possessed either a 'workhouse chair' or a 'shell', a type of stretcher, which was used throughout the parish as a form of ambulance to transport accident victims, or to move sick or immobile inmates. In this sense, unlike their 19th-century descendants, workhouses were highly integrated into local neighbourhoods rather than isolated from them. They were part of a range of sources of support that the disabled poor could choose to make use of (Hitchcock 2004, 132–49).

Conclusion

In a population of around nine million people at the end of the 18th century, probably only a few thousand people with physical or mental disabilities lived in some sort of institution. The medieval and early modern belief that care was the responsibility of family and the community persisted throughout the century. As the lives of disabled people, John Monro's casebook, Old Bailey trial records, and the narratives of the blind and deaf show, the vast majority of people with some sort of impairment, mental or physical, lived assimilated lives, largely accepted in their communities and integrated through marriage, kinship ties, work and the interactions of daily life. They were not seen as creatures of the institution, however poor, troubled or incapacitated they might be.

Imperceptibly though, the notion of the institution as the 'right place' for people who were seen as 'different' was beginning to insinuate itself into the public consciousness. A steadily increasing range of specialist buildings, or buildings used for specialist purposes, was in place. There were charitable hospitals, state military hospitals, institutions for the mentally ill, workhouses frequented by destitute disabled people, and specialist schools for blind and deaf children. Increasing state involvement in, and responsibility for, the lives of its citizens, particularly the poorest, was beginning to formalise and separate out types of need. The state, and the more influential citizens and reformers, began to seek rational, utilitarian responses to its problems, and disability began to be seen as a problem. The easy tolerance and acceptance that had characterised much of the 18th century began to dissipate.

As a new era beckoned, life for many disabled people was about to become very different indeed.

Discussion: Disability and charity

The long 18th century (the period from 1660 to 1820) saw the beginnings of a significant charity movement, part of which concerned itself with the lives of disabled people. What influence and impact has charity had on disabled people and attitudes towards them?

In 1990 a group of disabled people gathered in protest outside the ITV buildings in London where the annual Telethon was being recorded, a live televised fundraising event on behalf of people 'in need'. They carried hard-hitting placards with slogans such as: 'Telethon is a Pimp'; 'Is this a cripple-free zone?'; 'Apartheid Telethon'; and 'Ask us, Not Aspel' (Michael Aspel was a presenter of the televised event, who also hosted another programme called *Ask Aspel*). Their anger was about the non-inclusion of disabled people in this charitable spectacle ostensibly held on their behalf. They objected to what they saw as an affront to their own self-image, where they were portrayed as pitiable victims, who had no say in what was said about them or done for them.

Charity has always had this sort of double edge in relation to disabled people, as well as to other groups. While discernibly doing good work and raising funds without which people might experience hardship, there are times when charity is perceived as objectifying the very people it purports to support. As the American theorist Wolf Wolfensberger summarised in his description of the disabled person as an object of pity, 'the ... individual is seen as suffering ... and there is emphasis on alleviation of this suffering' and the 'individual is viewed with a "there but for the grace of God go I" attitude' (Wolfensberger 1975, 13).

Today our general understanding of the word charity, or charitable, is of kindness, a form of well-intentioned help and support for others in the face of difficulties. The word has not always held such positive connotations. In the 19th century the slang term 'cold as charity' reflected the unfeeling harshness with which charity was doled out to the 'unfortunate'. Charitable giving was also sometimes seen then as something to enrich the lives, or inflate the egos, of the donors more than a genuine engagement with or concern for those for whom money was being raised. A *Punch* cartoon in 1877 entitled 'Fashionable entertainments for the week' showed a monocled, top-hatted young man addressing an elegant young lady:

'Going to the Throat and Ear Ball, Lady Mary?'
'No – we are engaged to the Incurable Idiots.'
'Then perhaps I may meet you at the Epileptic Dance on Saturday?'
'Oh yes we are sure to be there. The Epileptic Stewards are so delightful.'
(quoted in Jarrett 2020, 162)

In much the same way, the Telethon protestors over a century later were accusing those involved in the event, and those promoting it, of being far more concerned with their own careers, social lives and public esteem than with those whose plight they were purportedly moved by.

In the 18th century, observers commented on the often-porous border between contempt and concern that could be at work in charitable giving to disabled people. Erasmus Jones, in a guide to urban etiquette in 1737, chided those who handed over alms to disabled beggars with no grace and with an element of judgement in their countenance:

Methought they did ill in doing good, and refus'd an alms while giving one. They seemed to insult over a poor creature's misery and seldom open'd their purse until they had vented their gall … There cannot be a greater mark of ignorance and ill manners than to gape at a person worn down in a consumption, afflicted with a jaundice, or labouring under any visible infirmity, as they pass along … because it oftentimes gives too great a shock to low spirits.

(Hitchcock 2004, 2)

Numerous motives can be at work in charitable giving. The great London military hospitals for disabled veterans were initiated by Charles II certainly in part because of his great rivalry with Louis XIV of France, who had recently initiated the construction of the splendid Hôtel des Invalides (literally 'House of the Disabled') in Paris. The aim of the charitable institutions was as much to show off the commercial wealth and military might and status of the great European states as to fulfil obligations to those who had become disabled fighting for their country.

The same could be said of many of the great institutions for the sick and disabled erected during the 17th and 18th centuries, such as the new Bethlem Hospital in London's Moorfields. They were signifiers of wealth and power – both of donors and of society as a whole – as much as they were receptacles of charitable aid for those who needed it. A charitable gift or legacy towards an almshouse, hospital or other institution worked as a marker of the donor's status, moral rectitude and success in the world. Charitable giving was a serious business – it has been estimated that the enormous total of £959,032 (well over 100 million pounds today) was given by Londoners for charitable purposes from 1601 to 1640 (Jordan 1960, 24).

In the medieval period charity was more closely tied up with notions of piety and religious salvation. Giving alms to disabled beggars was part of a litany of good works that might help pave the way to heaven for a sufficiently pious donor. Taking in destitute disabled people to the care of religious institutions was a charitable obligation for those who saw themselves as being on earth to carry out God's will. Establishing a charitable hospital for people with leprosy or others who were in need might ease the path through purgatory to eternal bliss, not only for the benefactor but also for important political figures they might wish (or need) to win over. In the 12th century William le Gros, Earl of Aumale (d 1179) undertook a deeply personal act of atonement, dedicating a handsome endowment of land, livestock and a hospital for 20 lepers. Beneficiaries of the endowment were asked to pray for the current King Henry II and his family as well as for the earl himself and his own family. As the historian Carol Rawcliffe has observed, his motives were a complex mixture of 'astute political calculation … anxiety about the afterlife and a desire to assist the needy' (Rawcliffe 2006, 105).

The disability activist and theorist Tom Shakespeare has noted that in more recent history 'one of the consistent themes in the British disability rights movement has been a vehement opposition to charities which claim to represent and support disabled people'. This theme was evident in the Telethon protests and also in the consistent tensions that have existed between disabled people and major charities such as Scope and Mencap. Shakespeare argues that while opposition to charity has played a powerful role in motivating disability activists and acted as a conduit for anger and frustration, the concept of charity upon which this is based is now somewhat outmoded. He claims that in today's world disability rights are not incompatible with charity, and that charities can play a role in removing the structural conditions, such as barriers to participation, which make people dependent on the generosity of others in the first place (Shakespeare 2006, 153–66).

Charity and disability have thus been locked in a complicated and uneasy embrace for many centuries. Who benefits most from charitable disbursements? Is it the disabled recipient whose life might be improved by a donation, or the giver, who might be motivated by pride, personal esteem, selfishness or even contempt for those to whom they give? Or is this too cynical a view of the charitable donor? Surely there are positive motivations also, of a genuine altruistic desire to support people who are perceived to be in need, to make society more inclusive and a better place to live for all its members?

At the heart of the current debate about charity is how to prevent the objectification of recipients of charity as perceived by the Telethon protestors, to ensure, echoing the slogan used by many disabled activists, that there should be 'nothing about us without us'. The question is also asked by some activists whether charity should have to be a factor in the lives of disabled people at all. It is argued that poverty and need are structural matters arising from a social system that excludes many disabled people from work or adequate benefit support. If this were to change, the need for charity would disappear.

Will it always be necessary for communities to offer financial support to their disabled members? The debate about charity and disability has not ended yet.

5 The 19th century: age of the asylum

Introduction and summary

If any period can be called the age of the institution for disabled people it is the 19th century. The appearance of England was changing dramatically as the Industrial Revolution gained pace and new towns, factories, railways and mills ate into the rural landscape. Alongside these changes came other new and strange sights.

Outside the towns and cities, there were the high walls and the towering chimneys of the county pauper lunatic asylum. 'From any of the great main lines of railway which run through the shire' proclaimed *The Builder* magazine in 1892, 'a traveller will be sure to spy, in some comparatively secluded position, a great group of buildings, which by their modern air … their tall chimney stacks and … their bulky water tower, seem to belong rather to the busy towns than to country seclusion'. This was the image of these new asylums that the average 19th-century person saw; something distant, something to marvel at, but not a place where they would ever wish to live themselves.

Then there were the monotonous, forbidding façades of the workhouses. In the years after the 1834 Poor Law Amendment Act, 350 of these were swiftly constructed at an average distance of 20 miles from each other. There had been workhouses previously, but of a more humane design and offering some assistance to the destitute disabled as well as services for the local parish. From 1834, the new workhouses were designed to punish the 'work-shy'. Soon many of them were not housing the non-disabled poor, who avoided them if they could, but disabled people and people who were mentally ill. With their spartan conditions and punitive work regimes, they were, intentionally, a miserable environment.

Why was there this great migration from the community into specialist buildings? At the beginning of the 19th century a few hundred people lived in nine small charitable asylums. By 1900 more than 100,000 'idiots and lunatics' were living in 120 county pauper asylums, with an average intake of almost 1,000. A further 10,000 were in workhouses.

Government and public attitudes hardened over this period. Following the French Revolution in 1789, amid fears that something similar might occur in England, the more laissez-faire attitudes of the 18th century were superseded by a less tolerant outlook. Those who stood out as different – including disabled people and those labelled mentally ill or 'idiotic' – were treated more warily, seen increasingly as a potential threat to social order and discipline. There was a political and religious drive to clean up the streets, to reclaim orderliness and stability from the unregulated chaos of the previous century. Even political radicals and revolutionaries were wary of the disabled, who did not fit well within their utopian quest for the perfection of society and humankind.

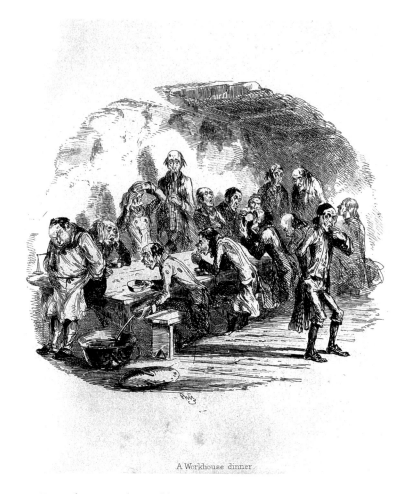

Fig 5.1
In the 19th century disabled
people began to drift into
workhouses.
[From *Sketches in London* by
James Grant. With twenty-
four humorous illustrations by
'Phiz'. Wellcome Collection.
Public Domain Mark]

A Workhouse dinner.

From the 1830s the workhouse was seen as a regime which would root out 'shirkers and scroungers'. No one should be given financial relief in their own home as this would make them lazy. Relief would only be given to the truly destitute, and it should take the form of a stay in a workhouse which they would be only too happy to leave (Fig 5.1). The impact this would have on the population of disabled people or mental illness was not foreseen.

The asylum, by contrast, was seen by some as a haven of peace, tranquillity and 'moral treatment' which would enable patients to recover. Others saw it as a repository which could shield society from its unwanted. A new class of medical professional, the 'alienist' (later to be known as psychiatrist), claimed that interventions in the asylum would cure and restore. But by the end of the century any early optimism of the alienists had changed to pessimism. Most people were deemed 'incurable' and never left the asylum, now seen as a building of containment for 'chronic' and dangerous cases (Fig 5.2). New modes of thought such as eugenics, which sought to perfect humans through better breeding and eradicate the 'defective', were a sinister augury of a new, darker era for disabled people.

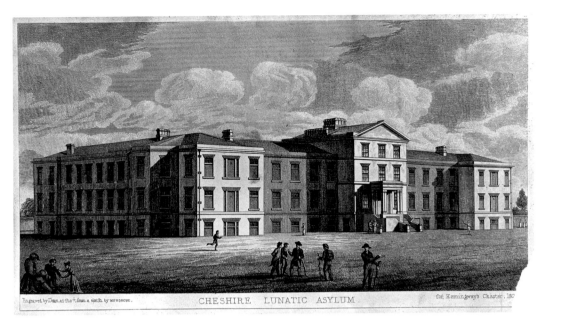

CHESHIRE   LUNATIC   ASYLUM .

Fig 5.2
Cheshire County Lunatic
Asylum in the 1830s.
[Line engraving by Dean
after Musgrove. Wellcome
Collection. Public Domain
Mark]

Even as these great shifts took place, many disabled people somehow remained in their communities. Accompanying the growth of asylums and other buildings was a rise in special educational provision and an explosion in charitable organisations and activity aimed at disabled people. While some begged on the streets, others prospered. The blind Henry Fawcett became postmaster general in 1880. Young disabled people sought to express themselves as worthy and contributing members of society. Members of the 'Guild of the Brave Poor Things' had as their coat of arms a sword crossed with a crutch. The battle for respect and acceptance continued in the face of an assault by those who saw no place in society for disabled people.

The birth of the public asylum

The advent of mass asylum building in the 19th century indicated a transformation in notions of correct treatment and care for those with mental illness and those deemed 'idiotic'. It also had major implications for deaf and blind people and those with physical disabilities, who could be caught up in the mass incarceration of those designated unable to cope. Up to this point it had been accepted in English society that disabled people or illness who needed care and support received it from family, friends and community. There was widespread acceptance of the idea that they should live within those communities, and to the fullest possible extent make their own way in life with the help of whatever family or social network they had around them. Only in the event of extreme destitution would the state, usually in the form of the local parish, or charity, intervene in their lives. Institutions were seen as neither solutions nor cures for a person's condition. This was to change radically as reformers, ostensibly benign and claiming to work in people's best interests, asserted that an asylum would be a safe place where 'lunatics' could be cured and 'idiots' taught, and where both groups could be controlled.

There were only nine voluntary, charitable institutions for 'lunatics' at the beginning of the 19th century. However, as the asylum movement gathered momentum, a relentless programme of asylum building would quite literally transform the English landscape. It would also bring about deep changes in public attitudes and social policy towards those deemed incapable of fitting in because of their troubled or supposedly under-developed minds. The 'mentally unsound' were moved in ever greater numbers from their communities to these proliferating institutions. Reformers claimed that those whose minds were disturbed or lacked capacity were unable to cope within modern society, and needed a professionally managed, self-contained, curative environment in which their senses could be restored and health improved to the point where, with luck, they could return to their homes. It was also pointed out that some lunatics could be a danger to others as well as to themselves, and that their unpredictable furies and irrationality were best safely contained and managed behind high institutional walls. It was the job of an expanding centralised state, which marked a departure from freewheeling 18th-century local parish management of local problems, and which was taking an increasing role in the regulation of the lives of its citizens, to attend to these problems. What was needed, it was commonly believed, was state-supported asylums.

Reformers were inspired by the example of the Quaker York Retreat, which had been established in 1796. The York Retreat was modelled on a 'mild system of treatment', doing away with the physical restraints that characterised institutions such as Bedlam and some madhouses, and offering instead kindly but firm interventions and management that aimed to restore a person's rationality. The idea was that the person would be encouraged to collaborate with the asylum in their own return to reason (Scull 1980). In this way the provision of more asylum treatment was presented as a liberal reforming cause that would undo the outrages of corrupt madhouses and put an end to Bedlamite horrors. However, the effect of such a humanitarian drive was to draw far greater numbers of people previously untouched by any notion of incarceration and separation from society into the institutional orbit. This was an integral part of the initiative to restore discipline and good order to society after the unregulated disorder, as reformers characterised it, of the 18th century, and in the face of the threats to social cohesion in England posed by the revolution across the channel in France.

Reflecting this growing government interest in mentally disordered individuals, there were parliamentary committees in 1807 and 1815. In 1808 the County Asylums Act was introduced. This was 'permissive' legislation which allowed local authorities to levy rates to fund the building of county asylums if they wished. In 1815, in an attempt to speed up the building process, further legislation was introduced allowing counties to borrow money to establish new asylums. The target population for these new institutions was 'pauper lunatics', meaning the poor, in contrast to the generally more well-heeled and privately funded occupants of the madhouses. Twenty new asylums were built as a result of the 1807 and 1815 legislation.

In 1845 a new and more comprehensive County Asylums Act *mandated* counties to build asylums to provide accommodation for all their pauper lunatics. A Lunacy Commission was established in the same year under the Lunacy Act to monitor them. One of the tasks of the Lunacy Commission was to ensure, in the spirit of the Poor Law Amendment Act of 1834, the transfer of all pauper lunatics from outdoor relief (that is, support in their own homes) and workhouses to specialist lunatic asylums.

New buildings sprang up at breakneck pace. By the end of the century there were as many as 120 asylums in England and Wales housing more than 100,000 people. In 1844 there had been 20,809 certified lunatics; by 1904 that number had multiplied more than five times, to 117,200, while the general population had merely doubled in the same period. The first 10 asylums built after the 1808 Act, such as the Cheshire County Asylum, housed on average 115 patients each. By the mid-1840s the average size for an asylum was 300 patients, with some, such as the Hanwell Asylum in Middlesex, housing as many as a thousand (Scull 1980, 48). Towards the end of the century, new buildings, such as the state imbecile asylums at Leavesden and Caterham outside London, were designed for 1,000 patients and soon became crowded with up to 2,000.

There were three main types of asylum. The 'conglomerate', a hodgepodge of miscellaneous structures (such as Suffolk County Asylum), the 'corridor' type, with wards connected by corridors up to a quarter of a mile long (for example Colney Hatch in Middlesex), and later the 'pavilion' type, with rows of female and male blocks each housing 150–200 patients (such as Leavesden Imbecile Asylum near Watford). Styles ranged from classical Greek to Gothic (Scull 1980, 50–4).

Entering though the large gates past the porter in his lodge, the visitor's eye would be caught by the looming water tower at the centre of the grounds, and the chapel. Clustered around the tower were the kitchens, laundries, workshops, recreation hall and administration block. On either side were the wards, with the sexes rigorously separated. Each ward housed up to 100 people. As many as 50 patients slept in one dormitory, their beds close together. They had day rooms for relaxation and large communal dining halls. Male and female attendants, as strictly segregated as their patients, worked and lived their lives on the site, often for generations (Scull 1980, 50–4).

Architecture played a central role in the policy of incarceration, isolation and restriction (Fig 5.3). Each asylum was designed with maximum security in the form of high surrounding walls and lockable wards and outer gates. There was ample ventilation, efficient drainage and optimal visibility of all patients to ensure a self-sustaining ecosystem of patient confinement. Buildings were designed to ensure efficient classification and segregation of different 'grades' of lunacy and idiocy, men and women, curables and incurables, the violent and the peaceful, the clean and the dirty. Everything was calculated to hinge around the four utilitarian principles of order, economy, efficiency and discipline (Porter 1992, 297).

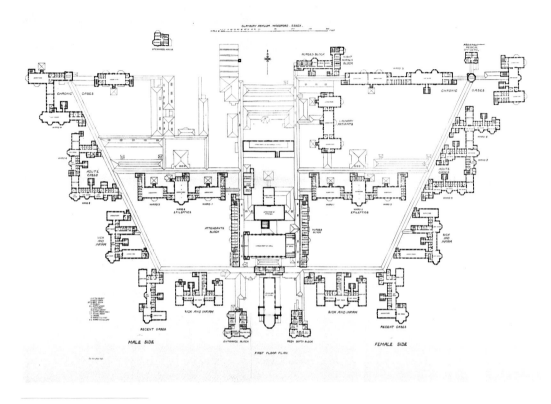

Fig 5.3
Architecture played a central
role in the incarceration of
patients.
[*Hospitals and Asylums of the
World* by Henry C Burdett
(1891). Wellcome Collection.
Public Domain Mark]

Asylums were a self-contained world in their rural settings. Their grounds were designed by some of the finest landscape gardeners. High walls prevented escape. The grounds contained farms, orchards, workshops, bowling greens, croquet lawns and cricket pitches. Walled gardens with shelters where patients could safely exercise, known as 'airing courts', led off the wards. There was always a cemetery. Some asylums even had their own railway stations, with a branch line into the grounds. The five asylums known as the 'Epsom cluster' in Surrey had their own light railway and rolling stock. There would often be an asylum fire brigade, with its own fire engine (Rutherford 2010, 22–24).

The number of people certified as 'insane' soared. The asylum created demand for its own services. Fewer and fewer people ever left, and more and more arrived. Over the century average asylum occupancy moved from 115 people to over 802 by 1900 (Porter 1992, 294). A great incarceration had taken place. Whatever earlier optimism there might have been that people could be cured in these ostensibly idyllic surroundings and then move on disappeared. The asylum became simply a place of confinement. New wings and storeys were constantly added until eventually a second or even third County Asylum had to be built in many areas. In London there were 11. In 1866 the physician Sir George Paget hailed the asylum as 'the most blessed manifestation of true civilization the world can present'. More than 125 years later, one historian described them as 'museums for the collection of the unwanted'

(Scull 1993, 267–333). The strange parallel world of the asylum has always stirred strong emotions.

Daily life in the asylum

One day in 1854, most of the 298 'lunatic and idiot' patients of the Norfolk County Asylum assembled in the grounds. It was time for drill. Responding to barked commands from nursing staff, they marched around the 30 acres surrounding the asylum. All of this was performed in front of the visiting lunacy commissioners. 'Great control is gained over the patients', commented a clearly impressed lunacy commission inspector, 'and the task of taking a vast number … for air and exercise becomes comparatively easy' (quoted in Roberts nd).

The asylum day was long, rigorously organised and highly controlled. At the Liverpool Asylum the bedroom doors of patients were unlocked at 6.00 am. Patients were washed, their hair brushed and the state of their skin examined. At 9.00 am, following breakfast, they were to be taken to the 'airing courts' and gardens while the wards were cleaned. At the Buckinghamshire County Asylum the focus was on work, preferably out of doors. For the men it was gardening and husbandry, for the women 'occupations suited to their ability', such as light hoeing and sorting potatoes (The National Archives, MH51/44B).

At the first Middlesex Asylum in Hanwell, London, patients were encouraged to keep small allotments to aid recovery. On the adjacent canal, produce from the asylum gardens was loaded onto barges at the 'asylum dock' and shipped to the London markets to generate income. Asylum diet could be better than in many working households, with fish or meat and vegetables for lunch, and bread and cheese supplemented by beer, cocoa and tea. Bedtime was at 8.00 pm, with long rows of beds two and a half feet apart. Many asylums had artisan workshops where men and women, strictly segregated, could work at different trades or occupations. There were workshops in which men could work as tailors, shoemakers, upholsterers, carpenters and blacksmiths. Women worked in the laundries and kitchens or did needlework for patients' clothes (Rutherford 2010, 36).

In 1851, the year of the Great Exhibition, Prince Albert opened the second Middlesex County Pauper Lunatic Asylum in Colney Hatch, north of London. With its Italian style, six miles of corridors and capacity for 1,000 people, it was the very model of modern asylum design. It had its own gasworks, brewery, farm and even an aviary breeding canaries. Its catchment area was north and east London. Within 15 years, 2,000 people were living there, including many from the large, impoverished Jewish community in London's East End. A kosher kitchen was installed and a Jewish cook employed. An interpreting attendant was recruited for the many Yiddish speakers. Craft workshops were managed by local artisans. Patients' boots and clothing and staff uniforms were made on site in tailoring workshops. There was also bookbinding, carpentry and mat making, and 150 women worked in the laundry. Patients kept canaries as pets and cats roamed the estate, used as vermin hunters. Within 50 years Colney Hatch had become effectively a small, overcrowded, segregated,

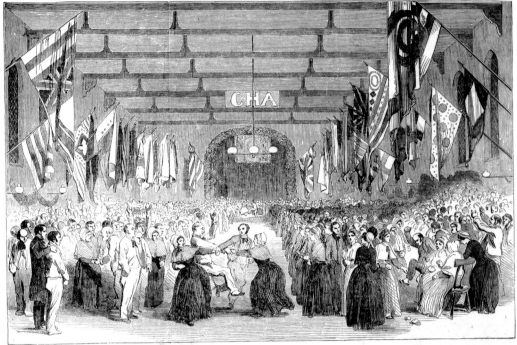

ENTERTAINMENT TO THE PATIENTS, AT THE MIDDLESEX COUNTY LUNATIC ASYLUM, COLNEY HATCH.

Fig 5.4

Having a ball? Entertainment for the patients at Colney Hatch asylum, in London, 1853.

[Wellcome Collection. Public Domain Mark]

enclosed town, with all the bustle and drama of the multicultural London streets that supplied it with its patients (Rutherford 2010, 17–18; Reeves 2011) (Fig 5.4).

Life had its own daily and seasonal rhythms. At the Buckinghamshire Asylum the chaplain would perform the Church of England service every Sunday, Christmas Day and Easter. There were Christmas parties and patient dances. Institutions even marked their own histories – the Sussex asylum celebrated its fourth anniversary with a grand ball in 1863 (The National Archives, MH51/44B). Recreation was provided which, although strictly regimented and usually confined within the asylum walls, marked asylum regimes out as less punitive than workhouses and prisons. In the better asylums reading was encouraged and newspapers were provided. Female patients were encouraged to crochet and knit and there were board games. Patients were encouraged to get outside as much as possible and to walk and take exercise in the airing courts, or the wider grounds, as fresh air was believed to be restorative to mental health. Sometimes croquet, skittles, quoits, bowls, tennis and badminton were played, and patients could be instrumental in constructing football and cricket pitches (Rutherford 2010, 38–9).

Asylums were, therefore, in a strange way, a replica, a specially constructed microcosm, of the outside world the patients had left behind. It mirrored that other world, but in so doing emphasised its separation and isolation from it. Asylum superintendents went to great lengths to recreate the outside world in artificial form. At the Normansfield Training

Institution for Imbeciles in Teddington just outside London, a replica West End theatre was meticulously created where the so-called imbecile patients could perform or watch productions. Dr John Langdon Down, the 'discoverer' of what is now called Down Syndrome, founded the private Normansfield institution and was its first medical superintendent. He saw the theatre – constructed at great expense – as a key element of the humane training and educational regime at the hospital. Yet it emphasised the separation of its inhabitants from any involvement in the world beyond the institution. It was never considered that the imbecile inmates might take the short train ride to visit an actual West End theatre – better to build them their own, however much that might cost, which only they and those who supervised them would attend (Fig 5.5).

It was also the case that asylums often fell far short of the places of humane treatment, recreation and restorative cure they purported to be. The optimistic forecast of health restoration and prompt return to the community of those who had been treated turned out to be an illusion. Discharge levels fell, and more and more patients became long-stay inhabitants of the asylums, seen as incurable. Over time the institutions became blocked up with masses of these so-called incurable patients, and no matter how quickly new asylums were constructed, overcrowding, demoralisation and bleak regimens of discipline and under-activity set in. The collapse of pretentions to provide cure was accompanied by the physical and moral decay of the asylums (Scull 1993, 269–77). In the

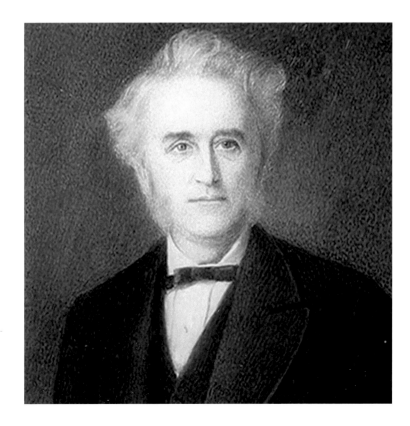

Fig 5.5
John Langdon Down.
[Sidney Hodges, c 1870.
St George's University of
London]

1870s the asylum investigator Mortimer Granville commented on the Colney Hatch asylum, such a flagship when opened by Prince Albert in 1851, as follows:

> Colney Hatch is a colossal mistake … it combines and illustrates more faults in construction and errors of arrangement than it might have been supposed possible in a single effort of bewildered or misdirected ingenuity … the wards are long, narrow, gloomy, and comfortless, the staircases cramped and cold, the corridors oppressive, the atmosphere of the place dingy, the halls huge and cheerless. The airing courts, although in some instances carefully planted, are uninviting and prison-like.
>
> (quoted in Scull 1993, 277)

Critics issued excoriating condemnations of asylum regimes, which they saw as having deteriorated to little more than regimented monotony,

> very well suited to a workhouse, but totally unfitted to an asylum for mental cure. Individuality is totally overlooked: indeed the whole asylum life is the opposite of the ordinary mode of living of the working classes. When the visitor strolls along the galleries filled with listless patients, the utter absence of any object to afford amusement or occupation strikes him most painfully. It is remarked with infinite approval now and then by the Commissioners that the walls have been enlivened with some cheap paper, that a few prints have been hung in the galleries, that a fernery has been established – matters all very well in their way, but utterly inadequate to take the place of the moving sights of the outside world.
>
> (Wynter 1870, 223)

And yet the bands played on. Asylum bands, as was the case with the band performing at the Norfolk Asylum for the visit of the lunacy commissioners, were quite common in the larger asylums. They were usually made up of both (male) patients and staff, and marched as they played their pipes and drums. This had a number of purposes. In part they were to replicate the situation outside. Victorian society became increasingly militarised as the century progressed, and marching bands were, among other things, a display of patriotism and of Britain's imperial strength and power. Many working men's institutions, workplaces, youth groups, church groups and others had bands whose processions were a common sight on the nation's streets. Asylum bands mirrored this, but were also seen, as the lunacy commissioners commented, as a form of both discipline and exercise. Patients would be marshalled to march in good order to the beat of the drums.

The Asylum for Idiots at Earlswood in Surrey had a particularly active band. Opened in 1855, Earlswood was the world's first purpose-built asylum for 'idiot children', entirely charitably financed (Fig 5.6). Its most famous superintendent was John Langdon Down, before he moved to establish Normansfield. Fully uniformed, Down's Earlswood band performed not only within the walls of the asylum but, unusually, outside. Marching was introduced for all male patients, and drills took place throughout the week, accompanied by the band with their drums, brass and pipes. In 1869 a group of 273 young idiots was escorted from

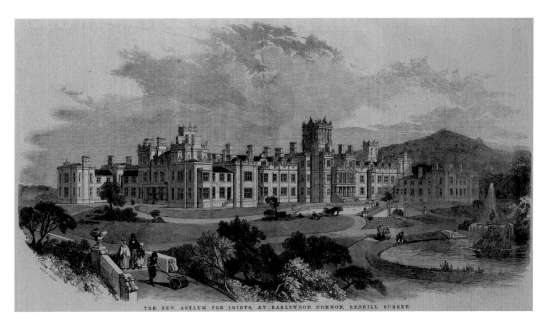

THE NEW ASYLUM FOR IDIOTS, AT EARLSWOOD COMMON, REDHILL, SURREY.

Fig 5.6
Earlswood, the world's first
purpose-built asylum for
'idiots' in the 1860s.
[Edmund Evans]

Earlswood to Brighton by train, where all the males marched behind the
band along the sea front. People who a century earlier had lived almost
unnoticed within their communities were now being displayed to the
British public as something strange and exotic, an unfamiliar spectacle to
be gazed at (Jarrett 2020, 213–15).

Momentous national events were celebrated. The coronation of
George V, Victoria's grandson, took place on 22 June 1911. The First
World War was just three years away. At the Western Counties Idiot
Asylum at Starcross, near Exeter, the day began with the inmates
performing a 'Trooping the Colour' spectacle. After a day of celebration,
as night drew in, the buildings of the asylum were illuminated and a flag
drill was performed, accompanied by the fifes and drums of the asylum
boys' band (Gladstone 1996, 154).

The asylum movement, despite the segregation and, often, the
depredations it imposed on those in its care, was in robust institutional
health, and had a further seven decades of life in it yet.

Public perceptions of disability – from Poor Law to eugenics

Public understandings of disability underwent a number of radical
transformations in this period, which marked a significant break with
the more easy-going and tolerant, if neglectful, attitudes of the 18th
century. A harsher tone set in, arising in part from political anxieties
about revolution, unrest and threats to the social order. There was a
feeling after the Napoleonic wars and the periods of economic depression
that subsequently took place that expenditure on poor relief was out of
control. Outdoor relief – supporting destitute people to continue to live
in their own homes with cash and in-kind relief such as clothing or food –

came to be seen as unfairly rewarding the work-shy and penalising those who looked after themselves. Disabled people continued to be seen, on the whole, as the 'deserving' poor in contrast to the allegedly feckless non-disabled who 'chose' not to work. However, they became much more an object of pity and charity, perceived as a problem that needed to be dealt with, rather than people who could be just left to themselves with a minimum of necessary support.

There was also a feeling that those who stood out as different from a perceived norm were a form of threat to social stability and cohesion. Politically, a level of conformity was seen as a requirement for belonging, and those who deviated radically in their political and religious beliefs or who had 'different' bodies or minds carried with them a sense of threat to social order. Removal from society was seen as an option for those who did not sign up to, or conform to, its precepts, as part of a wider campaign to clean up immorality and unrestrained social behaviour, and to restore communal order and discipline.

This ambivalent perception of disability, where a person was seen either as an object of pity or a matter of concern, was reflected in wider cultural representations. In the novels of Charles Dickens, for example, disabled characters ranged from the passive, almost comically sentimentalised Tiny Tim in the 1843 novella *A Christmas Carol* to the appalling dwarf character Daniel Quilp in *The Old Curiosity Shop* (1840), a monstrous villain who beats his wife and swindles everyone he meets (Figs 5.7 and 5.8). People's disabilities were always a matter of concern, never an incidental feature of who they were.

This estrangement of disabled people from society gathered pace with the anxieties generated by evolutionary theory, after the publication of Charles Darwin's *Origin of Species* in 1859. Darwin's work shocked Victorian Society in arguing that the human species had evolved, through a process of adaptation to its environment, from earlier species and, originally, a single organism lurking in a primeval swamp. It was only those species most fit for their environment, and most able to adapt to it, that survived (Fig 5.9). This undermined prevailing Christian beliefs that humans were created by God in his image to be a unique and dominant species on earth. Humans were closer to other animals than they would like to think, and perhaps not as special as they had imagined.

Fig 5.7

Dickens gave a cloyingly sentimental depiction of disability with his character Tiny Tim …

[Fred Barnard]

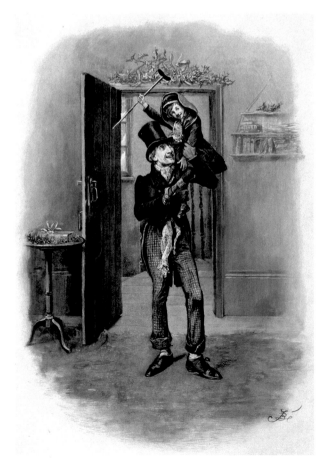

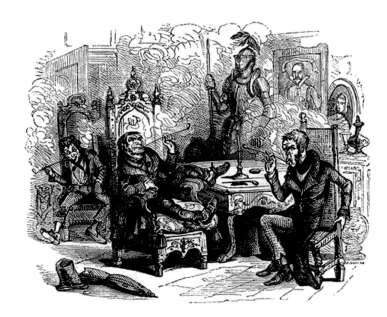

Fig 5.8
... but depicted the dwarf
Daniel Quilp as a monstrous
being in *Old Curiosity Shop*.
[Hablot Knight Browne]

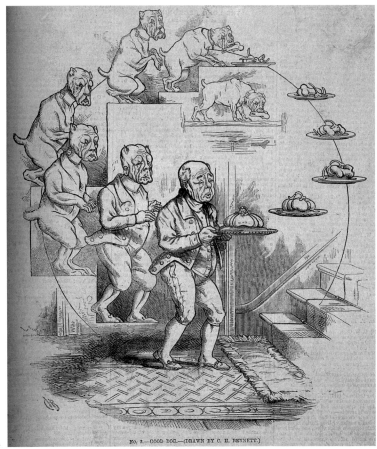

NO, 3.—GOOD DOG.—(DRAWN BY C. H. BENNETT.)

Fig 5.9
Darwin's theory of evolution
caused concern about the
bestiality of humans, and
was instrumental in the
emergence of eugenic science.
[Wood engraving after C
Bennett, 1863. Wellcome
Collection. Public Domain
Mark]

Darwin's work was adapted by his half-cousin Francis Galton into the science of eugenics (meaning in Greek 'good birth'). In his books *Hereditary Genius: An Inquiry into its Laws and Consequences* (1869) and *Inquiries into Human Faculty and its Development* (1883) he argued that heredity rather than environment was largely responsible for human differences. He advocated a national policy of social engineering to eradicate mental and physical disability and other human frailties (Fig 5.10). Eugenic scientists argued that a process of degeneration occurred through 'bad breeding' in a population. They blamed disability of all sorts (and poverty, prostitution, crime, alcoholism and immorality) on unrestrained breeding by the lower orders. The only way that degeneration could be reversed and the human stock improved, ensuring the survival of the race, would be to reduce breeding by the lower orders and increase reproduction in the middle and upper classes. Reducing breeding in the lower orders could be achieved by a range of interventions, including contraception, sterilisation, institutionalisation and even active euthanasia of the severely disabled.

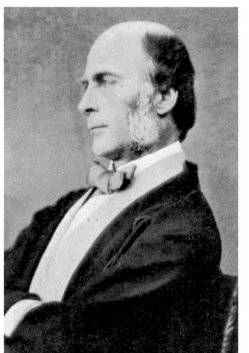

Eugenics was of course a deeply flawed mode of thought which barely deserves the name of science and it is now widely discredited (although its shadow survives in scientific developments such as gene therapy and prenatal testing). It took no account of environmental and social factors, accident, or chance in the causes of disability, and it chose to studiously ignore the incidence of disability in the middle and upper classes, which was of course widespread. However, it was widely adopted and believed by the intellectual classes, whose prejudices about the lower orders (however enlightened they imagined themselves to be) it fuelled. The effect of eugenic science was to demonise disabled people, to give spurious scientific authority to an idea that already existed in 19th-century society that somehow they did not belong. They became a mark of degeneration, a visible reminder that there was a threat to the survival of human society unless action was taken to improve the human stock and drive out weakness, disease and disability. Disabled people were seen as a brake on the progress of the rest of the population.

Fig 5.10
Francis Galton, who developed the pseudo-science of eugenics.
[Wellcome Collection. Attribution 4.0 International (CC by 4.0)]

This view, though fashioned from the secular theory of evolution and natural adaptation, carried striking echoes of earlier views of disability as a mark of sin or divine displeasure.

Eugenics influenced the thinking of many reformers and charity activists, almost all of them members of the middle or upper classes, who in general adopted a harsh attitude towards people living in poverty or with disability. The Charity Organisation Society (COS), which worked closely with Poor Law commissioners, was nicknamed 'Cringe or Starve'. They saw their role as the differentiation of the hard-working and deserving poor, who could be helped out of poverty by an injection of small amounts of relief, from the feckless, who should be condemned to a life of self-imposed destitution. With disability seen as a sign of the moral failures of a long line of previous generations or a consequence of a person's immoral and dissolute lifestyle, there was little encouragement for the mentally or physically disabled poor. Their problems related to their disability were too often seen as a matter of personal moral responsibility. Consignment to an institution was generally seen as the best option for them to live out the rest of their life of misfortune.

Workhouses

The nature of the workhouse changed suddenly and rapidly with the introduction of the Poor Law Amendment Act in 1834 and it became a very different place from the more relaxed environment of the 18th-century poorhouse.

The idea of this new legislation was that the 'idle' would be made to work in the workhouse. The system would be deliberately harsh with minimum comfort (chairs were to be made backless, to avoid ease of sitting), basic diet and separation of the sexes. Husbands and wives would live apart, as would parents and children. The theory was to punish the work-shy so that only the truly destitute or incapable would accept relief. In the five years after the Act, some 350 new workhouses were constructed, at a distance of roughly 20 miles from each other. A further 200 were built before the end of the century. The architects George Gilbert Scott and William Moffatt criss-crossed the country on horseback in the 1840s, picking up workhouse commissions. Their designs, based on standard model plans, excluded any sort of extravagance, were sited on the edges of towns to avoid offence to the citizens, and aimed for a standard below the average labourer's cottage, so as not to be too attractive to the destitute. Segregation was strict, diet meagre, work punitive (May 2011, 9–14) (Fig 5.11).

The consequence was that soon many workhouses were housing not the non-disabled poor but the old, the sick, the mentally ill and those with physical or learning disabilities deemed unable to work. In 1835 the Birmingham workhouse established purpose-built wards for 'insane' residents. The Leicester workhouse segregated 'idiots and lunatics', providing specialised nursing attendants. By 1837 more than 8,000 'idiots and lunatics' were under the care of parishes (Wright 2001, 15, 17–20). Workhouse staff struggled to care for them. In 1854 the master of the Southwell workhouse, Nottinghamshire, complained about a suicidal lunatic resident. The only way they could control the 'poor creature', he claimed, was to beat him around the toes and the head with a stick (The National Archives, MH12/9530/338).

An 1867 enquiry into London workhouses by the renowned medical journal *The Lancet* was highly critical of the accommodation and treatment of lunatic and idiot patients within the workhouse system. The investigators found one woman 'wandering up and down in a state of mingled frenzy and exhaustion. She had been admitted four days previously and had had no sleep since.' She had not eaten for four days. At the Chelsea workhouse they reported they had found that 'about thirty chronic insane patients wander in a melancholy, objectless manner about

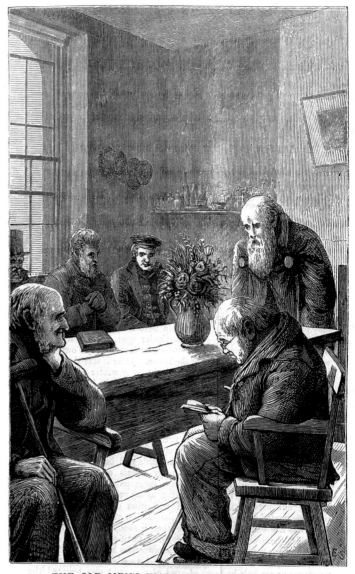

Fig 5.11
A depiction of a workhouse ward for old men, 19th century.
[Wellcome Collection. Public Domain Mark]

THE OLD MEN'S WARD IN THE WORKHOUSE.
XVI.–8.

the house and the yards' (Longmate 2003, 212–3). They found even worse at St Leonard's in Shoreditch:

> The general aspect of the wards is one of extreme cheerlessness and desolation … especially lamentable in the case of the lunatics and imbeciles. Moping about in herds without any occupation whatever, neither classified, nor amused, nor employed – congregated in a miserable day-room where they sit and stare at each other and at the

bare walls, and where the monotony is only broken by the occasional excitement due to an epileptic or the gibbering and fitful laughter of some more excitable lunatic.

(quoted in Longmate 2003, 213)

Physically disabled people also soon filled the bleak wards of the workhouses. One overseer wrote in 1851 about an infirmary ward at a workhouse which housed 'about 100 patients, the greater portion advanced in years, some stricken by the infirmities of age and nature, some lame and some blind'. They were all in a very hot and ill-ventilated toom at the top of the building where the windows could not be opened (Longmate 2003, 195). A visitor to the infirmary at St Giles workhouse in London in 1856 described it as follows:

> I had to wait with a crowd at the office door to obtain a ticket, visitors being allowed only for one hour once a week. The sick in the so-called infirmary, a miserable building ... were indeed a sad sight, with their wretched pauper nurses in black caps and workhouse dress. One poor young man there, who had lain on a miserable flock bed for fourteen years with a spine complaint, was blind: and his case would have moved a heart of stone; yet no alleviation of food or comforts was ever granted him, his sole consolation being the visits of a good woman, an inmate, who attended upon him daily, reading to him to while away the dreary hours.
>
> (quoted in Longmate 2003, 196–7)

His situation was not uncommon. The Workhouse Visiting Society's journal stated that 'it is no uncommon thing to find persons who have spent eight, nine or eleven years in one ward, or one bed'. They attributed this to the workhouse becoming a last resting place for those who either could not gain access to a hospital or could not be nursed at home (Longmate 2003, 197).

The sheer extent of the long-term occupation of workhouses by disabled and infirm people was made clear in an 1861 survey which estimated that around 20 per cent of workhouse inmates, or 14,000 people, had lived there for at least five years, 6,000 of them classed as 'old and infirm'. By 1863, in the 46 London workhouses, the vast majority of the inhabitants (90 per cent) were elderly, 'idiotic', blind or deaf and dumb (Longmate 2003, 197). This was recognised as a problem by government. From 1845 the newly established Lunacy Commission had been given powers to monitor the treatment of lunatics and idiots remaining in workhouses and to effect their transfer to publicly funded or charitable asylums.

In 1856 the Lunacy Commission commented that the huge insane wards in some workhouses were asylums 'in everything but the attendance and appliances which insure ... proper treatment'. But the asylum-building programme of the period was intended only for those who could be cured or who were disruptive. This excluded 'harmless and incurable idiots', 10,000 of whom remained in workhouses (Wright 2001, 17–20). Gruel, bread and cheese formed the diet, with soup or meat and potatoes once a week. Water was the only drink (with tea a privilege for

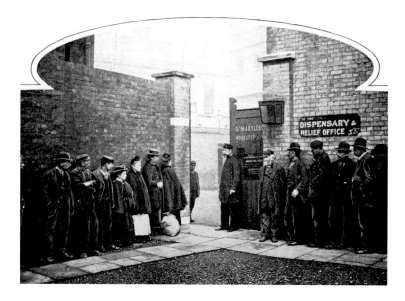

Fig 5.12
People queuing at St
Marylebone workhouse in
London at the end of the 19th
century.
[Wellcome Collection]

the elderly). Women made sacks or worked in the kitchen and laundry. Men chopped wood or ground corn (Englander 1998, 38–9).

The situation of disabled people in workhouses came to be seen as untenable, with people often neglected by drunk or incapable staff or brutally treated. The founding idea of the post-1834 workhouse, that through harsh institutional treatment the poor could be motivated to find work and return to their homes, proved to be utterly fallacious. The assumption that poverty was somehow self-inflicted took no account of the unavailability of work during times of economic hardship, nor did it acknowledge the destitution that could be brought on by disability. The effect was to fill workhouses with destitute people who were disabled, infirm, aged or lacking family support, imposing on them a punitive regime of bleak and joyless hardship (Fig 5.12).

Towards the end of the century efforts were made to reform workhouses and there was greater recognition that poverty and misfortune were caused by external factors beyond people's control rather than wilfully self-inflicted through idleness or fecklessness. Characters such as Dr Henry Bridges, who was appointed as medical inspector by the Poor Law Board in 1869, implemented much needed reforms to the infirmary sections and medical services provided under the workhouse system. He condemned the 1834 Poor Law as a 'gross insult to the people' (Longmate 2003, 209).

Despite their cruel reputation for their treatment of the poor, and their brutalising and disproportionate effect on the lives of the disabled poor, the workhouses survived. There were official attempts to move lunatics and idiots to more 'appropriate' asylum settings, but by 1906 there were still 11,500 people of 'unsound mind' in workhouses, which meant an average of 19 people in each workhouse. As late as 1914 there were 400 people certified as lunatics in workhouses in one part of Essex (Longmate 2003, 220). The last few workhouses would linger on until 1948, renamed as public assistance institutions.

Life in the community, education and charity

'Some boys laugh at poor cripples when they see them in the street', observed a religious advice pamphlet for children in 1848. 'Sometimes we meet a man with only one eye, or one arm, or one leg, or who has a humpback. How ought we to feel when we see them? We ought to pity them.' The writer had a sting in the tail for the jeering boys. While cripples might be made 'bright and beautiful' by God on judgement day, wicked non-disabled children who laughed at them could be 'burned in a fire that will never be put out' (Mortimer 1848). These were the ambivalent Victorian attitudes towards disability – a combination of fear, pity, discomfort and an underlying idea, familiar from previous centuries, that some form of either benign or malign divine judgement was at play. Were disabled people being punished by God in having disability visited upon them, or was it the non-disabled who were undergoing a divine test of their capacity for pity and compassion?

The pull of the asylum and the workhouse was strong, but many thousands of disabled people remained in their communities. Some lived in abject poverty. The social investigator Henry Mayhew described the disabled beggars of the London streets in 1862 (Fig 5.13), including the 'idiotic looking youth … shaking in every limb' or the 'crab-like man without legs strapped to a board (who) walks upon his hands'. He expressed surprise that there was 'no home or institution for cripples from this class. They are certainly deserving of sympathy and aid for they are utterly incapacitated from any kind of labour' (Quennel 1987, 404). He also recorded his encounters with clusters of 'imbeciles' as he walked through the lodging houses of the deeply impoverished St Giles area:

> Many of them were middle-aged men … very shabbily dressed, and some half-naked. There was little manliness left in the poor wretches … the inspector told us they were chiefly vagrants, and were sunk in profound ignorance, from which they were utterly unable to rise.
>
> (Quennel 1987, 175–6)

Other disabled people prospered or achieved fame. James 'Deaf' Burke (1809–45), also known as 'the deaf un', rose from poverty to become a world champion prize fighter. An illiterate orphan who haunted the London waterfront, his fighting talent was spotted and he quickly rose to prominence in the brutal, largely unregulated world of 19th-century boxing, in which fights could go on for over a hundred rounds and would usually last until one of the fighters had been battered into insensibility. He went to America where he introduced Prize Ring fighting, and fought in New York and New Orleans. Back in England he retired from boxing in 1840, aged 31. For a while he prospered as a stage actor advertising his magnificent physique, but a life of excessive drinking, womanising and poor diet brought him to a penniless death in 1845 (Jackson and Lee 2001, 30–1).

Henry Fawcett (1833–84) was blinded as a young man in a shooting accident during a partridge hunt. His blindness was an obstacle to his planned legal career and so he followed a more individual path, building a political career through writing, speaking and nurturing his public

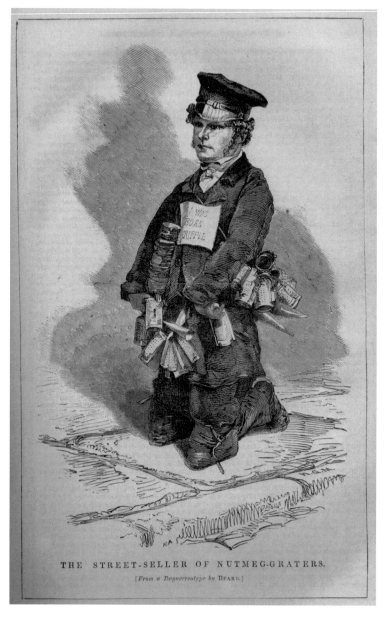

THE STREET-SELLER OF NUTMEG-GRATERS.

[From a Daguerreotype by BEARD.]

Fig 5.13
The street seller of nutmeg
graters, 1851.
[From Henry Mayhew's
London Labour and the London
Poor, 1851]

profile. He became a liberal MP in 1865, representing first Brighton and
later Hackney until his death in 1884. He was appointed as postmaster
general in 1880, where he was responsible for the introduction of the
parcel post. After his death from pneumonia aged just 51, something
approaching national mourning ensued, with tributes in Parliament, the
press and from the queen. Fawcett is said to have been the second most
popular man in England after the prime minister, Willian Gladstone. He
was certainly the most influential blind person of his time (Goldman
2006).

Educational provision for children and young disabled people grew rapidly. Literacy and education began to be considered (in some educational provision at least) equally important to traditional vocational training. In 1838 the London Society for Teaching the Blind to Read was formed. In 1866 the Worcester College for the Blind ('for the blind sons of gentlemen') became the world's first further education establishment for disabled people (Safford and Safford 1996, 126). After 1879 the Poor Law authorities were allowed to support institutions and societies caring for blind, deaf and dumb children, and from the 1890s this included day schools for 'defective' and epileptic children. By the late 19th century there were 50 blind institutions in Britain outside London educating 1,113 people, and 26 institutions for the education of over 2,000 deaf pupils. In 1897 these institutions were re-titled Royal Schools. By 1899 there were also 43 specialist schools in London (Borsay 2005, 94–6).

The general aim of such schools was 'trained adaptability' so that when children completed their education they could take advantage of whatever openings there might be. Children typically spent their days on communication (including braille or signing), mathematics and scripture, while there was also an emphasis on handicrafts and other practical skills. In most deaf schools, from the age of 12 boys took woodwork while girls did domestic science, laundry, cookery, housecraft and advanced needlework, including dressmaking. A debate raged across Europe about whether deaf education should be conducted through the oral medium (lip reading) or signing, and although in 1880 the World Congress to Improve the Welfare of the Deaf and Blind conference in Milan decided that 'only oral instruction could fully restore deaf people to society', 74 per cent of British schools supported sign language above the oral or combined method (Borsay 2005, 96–7).

The Victorian era also saw a huge explosion in charitable activity. By the end of the century there were hundreds of organisations providing community or institutional services to disabled people. In 1868 the British and Foreign Blind Association was formed by Dr

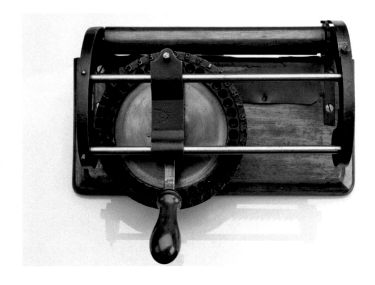

Fig 5.14
An early writing machine for blind people, a precursor to Braille, 1820s.
[Science Museum, London.
Attribution 4.0 International
(CC by 4.0)]

Thomas Armitage, initially to promote the use of Braille. It was to become the Royal National Institute for the Blind (Phillips 2006). There were charitable bodies for the blind, the 'deaf and dumb', 'lunatics', 'idiots', 'epileptics' and 'the deformed'. They offered education (The Association for the Oral Instruction of the Dumb), work (Liverpool Workshops and Home Teaching Society for the Blind), hospital treatment (National Hospital for the Paralysed and Epileptic) and many other services (Fig 5.14).

As this educational and charitable activity demonstrated, the asylum or other institution was not an inevitable destination. Many disabled people simply soldiered on purposefully in their communities. In 1894 the first branch of the Guild of the Brave Poor Things (motto 'Happy in my lot') was formed. This was ostensibly a self-help group for people with physical impairments, although they were dominated by formidable charitable pioneers, such as their founder Grace Kimmins in London, who were not disabled themselves but saw it as their life's work to help those less fortunate than themselves. They described themselves as a group to 'make life sweet for the blind and crippled folk of all ages'. Conveying a sense of pride and solidarity, they used popular military imagery of the period to create positive feelings about their disabilities, referring to themselves as 'a great army of suffering ones'. Their annual report in 1902 described how they 'go out daily into a battle-field, where pain is the enemy to be met and overcome' (Mantin 2009).

Outside the walls of the 19th-century asylum, the daily battles for survival, fame, or simple respect continued to be fought across the towns and cities of England.

Conclusion

The 19th century was a turning point for disabled people in English society. It was during this period that care for the individual disabled person substantively shifted from the family and community to the institution and the state. A number of factors caused this. There had been the steady growth of a small number of institutions which had accelerated towards the end of the 18th century, with reformers arguing that a quiet, isolated restorative environment was a better option for the mentally or physically disabled person than trying to cope with the demands and pressures of society. Such thinking gained wider acceptance as the 19th century progressed, influenced in part by growing urbanisation and industrialisation.

At the same time there was an increasing shift from highly localised parish administration to more centralised state control, and greater state and governmental interest in regulating the everyday lives of people. This led to more state-led approaches and interventions in anything perceived as a problem. Disability became problematised, seen as something which caused social anxiety and needed a solution in a way that had not been the case in smaller parish communities. Institutions began to be seen as the solution. The encouragement to build state-funded asylums from 1808, and the obligation to build them from 1845, were clear markers of this shift.

Previous attitudes of benign neglect and laissez-faire tolerance gave way to much harsher public, or certainly governmental, perceptions. The harshness of the 1834 Poor Law Amendment Act, fear of social unrest and even revolution, and anxieties about moral collapse all led to a framing of disability as either an object of pity or a signifier of dangerous difference. Either way, the disabled person came to be seen less and less as a person who belonged. The emergence of eugenic 'science' towards the end of the century embedded these harsh attitudes even more markedly, and disability came to be seen by many, certainly among the intellectual classes, as a moral failing and a panic-inducing symbol of social and moral degeneration.

However, the eugenicists, the institutions and the reactionary lawmakers were not the whole story. Many disabled people simply carried on in their communities as best they could, working if possible. Some, like the deaf boxer James Burke, achieved fame and popular renown; others like the blind postmaster general Henry Fawcett rose to the top in their chosen profession. Most simply lived their lives, proud of who they were and accepted by those around them, even as others tried to institutionalise them off the face of the earth.

Discussion: Myths and stereotypes

Early in the asylum era disabled people were portrayed as innocent and helpless, in need of protection. Later in the same era, they were portrayed as dangerous and threatening, and needing confinement. This raises the question of the differing ways that disabled people have been portrayed over time, and why these shifts in perception have occurred.

Perceptions of disability are complex, multifaceted and changing. Whenever we talk about a particular perception in a particular period by a particular group of people, we should remember that there are always countervailing viewpoints. One way of thinking about disability might be dominant at some point, but it is never the only way of thinking.

For example, during the period of eugenics from the late 19th century through to the Second World War (1939–45), it is certainly true to say that many intellectuals, politicians, policy makers and other influential people, across the political spectrum, signed up to the central assumptions of eugenics. They believed that disability represented an existential threat to the racial health of society and needed to be 'bred out' of the population, and even identified mental impairment (and some physical impairments) as the root causes of crime and violence. We can therefore speak of this period as the 'eugenic era'.

However, many people thought differently. The liberal MP Josiah Wedgewood, for example, spoke up against the 1913 Mental Deficiency Act (a piece of legislation long advocated by the Eugenics Society) on human rights and civil liberty grounds. The distinguished psychiatrist and geneticist Lionel Penrose despised eugenics, denounced its association with racial purification, and in his 1938 *Colchester Survey* debunked many of its precepts (Figs 5.15 and 5.16). We can also be sure that most disabled people did not perceive themselves as the threat that eugenics assigned to them, nor did their families and many members of the

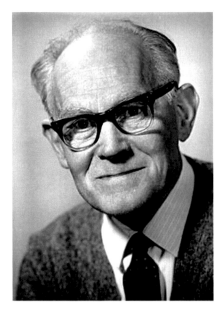

Fig 5.15
Lionel Penrose, who stood
firm against the tide of
eugenics.
[Godfrey Argent]

Fig 5.16
Josiah Wedgwood MP,
who opposed the Mental
Deficiency Act on human
rights grounds.
[Wikimedia Commons]

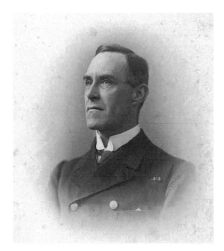

public, who would have been repelled by the vicious libel perpetrated against them. A perception can therefore be dominant, but is never unchallenged or the sole point of view.

As this book has argued, there have always been numerous explanations, understandings and theories of disability. In the medieval period it could be seen as both a gift or a punishment from God. It could be seen as taking a person closer to God through the suffering they shared with Christ, or as an exemplar of the consequences of sin (their own or other people's). It could also have naturalistic explanations or be seen in a medical context. In the 18th century the 'imperfection' of disability could be seen as God's work. Perfection could only be understood if there was imperfection against which it could be measured, so imperfection was just as important in the world as its opposite. Thinkers also argued that everything in the world was created by God and could not therefore be criticised, ridiculed or disrespected. All types of person had their place in the Great Chain of Being (as long as they knew it, and stayed where God intended them to be).

Asylums could be seen either as places of improvement, cure, education and restoration, part of an idealistic approach to solving complex social problems and injustices, or as dumping grounds, places of isolation for those who did not belong. While the 'therapeutic optimism' pole of this spectrum of opinion was probably in the ascendant in the early decades of the asylum movement, 'therapeutic pessimism' had achieved a dominant position by the time of eugenic science at the end of the 19th century. 'Cure' had not happened on the scale the optimists had envisaged and the asylum population grew exponentially, many confined for the rest of their lives once admitted. With this shift came a shift in rationale for the asylum and perceptions of disability. It was not to improve, educate and cure those who were admitted, it was to confine those who were a danger to themselves or others, to protect society from the threat they posed.

It was not disabled people who had changed over this period. It was the prevailing perceptions about them. In this sense we can talk about disability being constructed. While there is a bodily reality that disabled people experience, their identity as a disabled person is at least partly formed by the cultural and social environment within which they live. In this sense disability is not a universal unchanging idea over time, a stable concept, but rather a construct of time and place.

Of course, most people do not theorise intellectually about disability, they simply experience it as a disabled person or as someone who knows or is related to a disabled person. Day-to-day interactions and the negotiation of daily life are deeply pragmatic experiences for most people, which leave little space or time for theorisation and abstract concepts. Many of the examples in this book show such interactions taking place over many centuries. Disabled people have always been part of the fabric of the communities they live in and always will be. Nevertheless, ideas matter and can influence life experience, however removed they might seem from everyday life when they first appear. There can be large structural changes driven by certain modes of thinking, such as the closing down of religious centres of care during the English Reformation, the building of asylums 400 years later, or the closure of asylums and the return to 'care in the community' of the late 20th century.

There can also be more subtle but equally impactful influences on how people are able to live their lives. If there is a generally benign and accepting attitude to disability at certain times, people's lives can be less challenging than during eras of hostility in which hate crime, marginalisation and other abuses can flourish. The historical trajectory is not linear, progressing from a bad past to a better present. There are times in early history when disabled people have occupied an integrated and included place in society, while the most heinous crimes against them, such as eugenic exclusion and Nazi extermination, have occurred within living memory. Hate crime, discrimination and marginalisation can play just as big a part in the lives of disabled people today as they have in the past, however sophisticated the technology, however progressive the laws and charters of rights, however inclusive the philosophies.

Perception of disability is therefore of critical importance. As Wolfensberger and other theorists have pointed out, ostensibly benign ideas about disability, such as the person as an object of charity or pity, can be just as degrading as more visibly hostile perceptions such as the subhuman or the menace. What is always missing in these perceptions is the voice of the disabled person themselves. Instead, their value and their identity have been formed by the viewpoint of others, of the non-disabled. One of the positive developments of the late 20th century was the emergence of the disability movement, in which disabled people seized back their identities from those who sought to define them and projected their own image of themselves onto society. This was the struggle of those who protested outside patronising charity events such as Telethon, of those who fought medicalised power over disabled people, and those who battled for equal citizenship and rights. It was all, ultimately, about controlling and owning their own identity and self-perception, and discarding myths and stereotypes.

However, to bring the debate to one of its most recent iterations, Tom Shakespeare has argued that the time is now ripe, following these battles, to rethink identity and social model politics of disability and to move to a post-identity era, where disabled people seek what they have in common with non-disabled people, promoting inclusion and equal status, rather than separatism. The goal of disability politics, he claims, should be to make disability and impairment irrelevant wherever possible, and move away from separatist notions (Shakespeare 2014, 110). What place for myths and stereotypes in such a world?

6 War and peace, 1903–45

Introduction and summary

'What are we going to do? Every defective man, woman and child is a burden. Every defective is an extra body for the nation to feed and clothe, but produces little or nothing in return.' So wrote, in 1930, Julian Huxley, public intellectual, secretary of the London Zoological Society and chairman of the Eugenics Society. He was not alone. The eugenic ideas that had come into circulation at the end of the 19th century became pervasive in English public debate in the first half of the 20th. Many public figures embraced the idea of eugenics, the need to 'manage the human stock' and avoid, as birth control pioneer Marie Stopes called it, 'race suicide' (Fig 6.1). The aim – which appealed to the political left and right – was to strengthen the human race, eliminating physical and mental defects to build a better society. Human perfectibility was very much part of the currency of early 20th-century thought.

However, there was an uneasy tension between two ways of thinking about disability, as the legacy of the Victorian asylum era came up against the new realities of the 20th century. On the one hand there was the threat to the 'health of the nation' from anyone considered disabled or 'deficient'. This called for isolation and segregation. On the other hand, tens of thousands of newly disabled British ex-servicemen came home from the battlefronts of the First World War between 1914 and 1918 (Fig 6.2). The presence of these young men, who had sacrificed their bodies for the nation, demanded a different way of thinking. There was also a growing body of thought, led by the researches of a new breed of social 'investigators', that poverty and environment were often major causal factors in disability, not just heredity, or perhaps not heredity at all.

This sudden influx of newly disabled people had a profound impact on society's responses to impairment, and the urgency and seriousness with which they were put into action. There were improved prosthetic limbs and advances in plastic surgery. Exercise and fitness approaches to repair and rehabilitate both physical and mental damage were introduced. Employers were urged to accommodate disabled workers into their factories and businesses, and a network of

Fig 6.1
Birth control pioneer Marie Stopes saw 'defective breeding' as 'race suicide'. [Wellcome Collection. Attribution 4.0 International (CC by 4.0)]

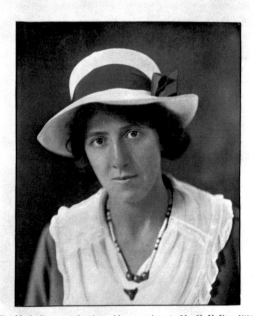

Dr. Marie Stopes at the time of her marriage to Mr. H. V. Roe, 1918.

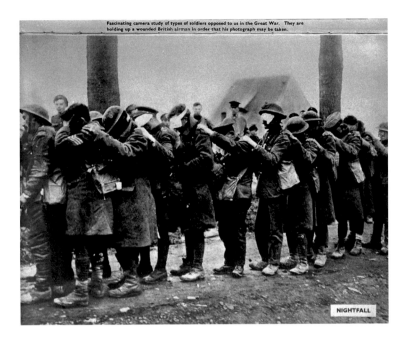

Fascinating camera study of types of soldiers opposed to us in the Great War. They are holding up a wounded British airman in order that his photograph may be taken.

NIGHTFALL

Fig 6.2
Blinded First World War soldiers. The First World War meant a huge influx of newly disabled people into British Society.
[Wellcome Collection. Attribution 4.0 International (CC by 4.0)]

sheltered employment initiatives sprang up, including the British Legion poppy factory in south London. New housing was built for disabled ex-servicemen, ranging from single cottages to entire special villages.

However, these changes did not always spread to the civilian disabled population. Those not disabled by war complained that they were treated like 'second-class' disabled people. To some extent, an exception to this could be found in heavy industries, such as coalmining, with a high incidence of disabling injuries. The labour movement in these industries introduced schemes to assist disabled union members through the provision of vital needs such as prostheses, insurance and sometimes rehabilitation and reintegration into the workforce. Nevertheless, unemployment among the civilian disabled population was sky-high in the 1920s and 1930s. While this added to the alienation and marginalisation of the population of people with physical impairment, for the 'mentally deficient' – people we would recognise today as having learning disabilities – ostracisation from society started to become total. A new network of 'colonies' was established. So-called mental defectives were a particular target of eugenic malice. The colonies were self-contained small worlds set in rural areas. As well as the 60-person 'villas' which housed the large numbers of men, women and children who lived there, there were farms, laundries, bakeries, recreation halls, chapels and mortuaries. Within this closed world, segregation by sex, age and ability was strict. Total separation from the outside world throughout life was the main aim.

Childhood disability was widely prevalent. Between 1900 and 1945 up to half a million children had some sort of physical disability or sensory impairment. Many of them were from the poorer working classes, the diseases and problems of poverty and the absence of immunisation contributing to the high prevalence of disability. Life

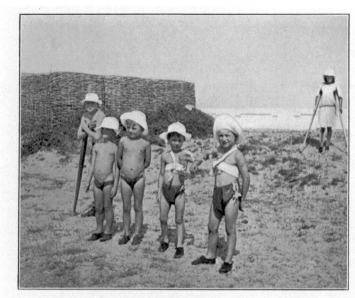

A Glimpse of Hayling.

Fig 6.3
Children from Lord Mayor
Treloar's Cripples Hospital
and College, 1937.
[Wellcome Collection]

both at home and at school could be difficult. Many families lacked resources for specialist equipment or treatment. Education became a right, but school regimes for 'crippled', blind and deaf children could be harsh and punitive, with low aspirations. However, some pioneered new approaches. These included progressive 'sunshine homes' for blind children and the phenomenon of the 'open air' school, believed to improve the health of disabled young people. Many children were trained only for low-skilled work, in the belief that they would be lucky to secure any sort of job at all (Fig 6.3).

A divide opened up in the understanding of mental illness, as medicine staked its claim to be the exclusive authority which could identify, diagnose, treat and control any form of mental disturbance. Mental illness came to be seen as a disease, or a range of diseases, treatable, once understood, by medical professionals in the form of drugs and physical interventions, in the same way as any bodily illness or malfunction. A challenge to this medical-scientific project came from the work of Sigmund Freud, who argued that mental disturbance had complex psychological roots, unconscious operations of the mind caused by childhood and other traumas. These could only be resolved through psychoanalysis, the talking cure, which would enable the patient to resolve their inner conflicts and return to a state of mental equilibrium.

Disability and children

How could high levels of disability among children in the early 20th century be explained? With eugenic thinking becoming a dominant factor in middle-class thought, and influential in policy circles, the 20th century opened as a difficult time for disabled people. Not only was there a feeling that disability of any sort was bad for the wellbeing of society, there was also an underlying, often unspoken, accusation that impairment was somehow the fault of the disabled person themselves, or of their parents. Behind all this was a generalised anxiety that the health of the British nation was declining and that this was manifest in high levels of disease, illness and disability, particularly among the poorest in society. High levels of childhood disability fuelled such eugenic anxieties. These fears were exacerbated by the poor physical condition of many young working-class recruits who volunteered to fight in the South African War (also known as the Second Boer War) of 1899. More than 35 per cent of volunteers were considered unfit for any type of military service, causing great public consternation (Anderson 2011, 16).

In opposition to eugenics there were more thoughtful understandings and explanations of disability, which had begun with some of the great social investigators such as Joseph Rowntree and Charles Booth from the late 19th and early 20th centuries. Such proponents rejected the idea that the poor had brought disability upon themselves through their own fecklessness. Their new explanations were based on empirical research carried out among poor communities. These evidenced that poverty, with accompanying neglect, poor housing and inadequate medical care were all instrumental in fuelling levels and incidence of disability. Poverty was not the result of idleness, but of wider social forces such as structural unemployment, over which people had no control.

Diseases that tended to ravage poor communities, such as rickets and tuberculosis (TB), were widespread. Rickets caused a softening of the bones resulting in bowed legs. It was caused by a lack of vitamin D, meaning that children in crowded, poor urban areas who lacked sufficient access to fresh air and exercise were particularly vulnerable. TB, also common in crowded, poor urban communities, as well as proving fatal for some, could attack the spine, hips and joints, adversely affecting mobility and weakening bones. Cerebrospinal meningitis, of which there was an epidemic in 1910, could cause deafness, as could measles and scarlet fever. Ophthalmia neonatorum, meaning conjunctivitis of the newborn, caused blindness in large numbers of new-born children (Anderson 2011, 17–18). All of these disabling diseases and conditions were far more common in areas of low socio-economic status than elsewhere. Much disability was a direct and visible consequence of poverty. It was certainly not a signifier of low morals, self-neglect and incapacity as eugenicists tried to argue.

As well as disease, working-class children were vulnerable to disabling injuries caused by dangerous environments in poor areas. In 1909 over 26,000 injuries were recorded from cars, which were becoming a new, largely unregulated and dangerous presence on the streets. As car ownership continued to rise, so did deaths and injuries from accidents. Most of the victims were pedestrians, and many injuries had disabling consequences. More than 180,000 traffic accident injuries were reported in the 10 years from 1927 to 1937. Around 14,000 children were killed in the same period. The urban playground of the streets in poorer areas was a danger zone for many, where death and disability could lurk (Anderson 2011, 18).

Disabled adults and employment

Self-evidently, large numbers of children with disabilities meant that a burgeoning population of adults would follow. For these, employment was a particular issue. Low expectations in the education sector, prejudice in employment practice, an absence of flexibility and adaptation in workplaces, and job scarcity combined to make access to employment extremely hard for disabled people. With minimal welfare support available at this time, there was a stark link therefore, as there had been in previous centuries, between disability, unemployment and poverty. A study conducted by the City of Birmingham Education Committee in 1911 demonstrated the overwhelming nature of the employment problem for disabled people. The report found that only 20 per cent of 'male cripples' were economically active, a situation exacerbated later in the century as the great depression struck in the 1930s (Borsay 2005, 129).

There were some efforts inside and outside government to address, or at least alleviate, these problems. The Workmen's Unemployment Act of 1905, implemented by a Conservative and Liberal Unionist coalition government, recognised that factors other than laziness and personal irresponsibility could cause unemployment. The Act authorised local Poor Law authorities to provide non-stigmatising jobs for those most vulnerable to unemployment, which included those 'unable to work at their trade due to old age, illness or some other misfortune'. Disabled people were included under the category 'some other misfortune' (Borsay 2005, 126).

The charitable sector led specialist employment initiatives, recognising the urgency and significance of the unemployment problem in relation to disability. This meant, however, that disabled people were highly dependent on the sector for work. From 1904 the National Institute for the Blind operated premises where blind masseuses practiced, and from 1916 an employment bureau for blind piano tuners. These were predicated on the belief that people lacking one sense often had heightened awareness and ability in their remaining senses, the enduring centuries-old idea known as the 'compensatory faculty'.

From the 1920s the Central Council for the Care of Cripples began working with adults as well as children, focusing on the formation of employment committees, which included employers and trade unions. Curative workshops, as they were known, were established to train disabled people in skills such as carpentry, joinery and shoemaking. The aim was not only to equip people with the skills they might need to enter or re-enter the workplace, but also to provide 'interesting labour' to overcome the despondency or depression that disability might cause (Borsay 2005, 129–31). Unemployment was not only instrumental in the extreme levels of poverty that many disabled people experienced, but also in marginalising and excluding them from having any stake, or sense of worth, in the society they lived in. Through collective self-organisation medical aid societies were formed.

Amidst mass unemployment there were many unsettling examples of how little incentive or motivation there was for employers to recruit disabled workers. A young man, Ron Moore, whose legs had been amputated after a road accident as a child, described his debilitating and demoralising search for a clerk's job in the 1930s:

> For six months I went day after day to banks and insurance offices in the City … Sometimes I managed to see the manager but I wasn't in very good shape by the time I got to the interview. The artificial legs rubbed blisters where they joined the tops of my legs and they often bled. It was very painful walking around so when I got to the manager's office I had to ask to sit down. That didn't make a very good impression because in those days you were expected to stand to attention, cap in hand. Well they always said the same thing. 'You've got no legs have you. I'm afraid we can't employ you.'
>
> (Humphries and Gordon 1992, 124–5)

As well as large numbers of people who had been disabled since birth or childhood, there was also a high incidence of acquired permanent disability in adulthood from workplace accidents. Many workplaces had minimal protections in place. Accidents largely occurred in working-class occupations, and the industrial workspace in particular was often a dangerous place. Mining was one of the most dangerous of all occupations. As well as accidents underground that caused disability, there was a risk of pneumoconiosis, a disabling lung condition caused by coal dust, and conditions such as 'beat' hand, knee or elbow, where swollen and infected skin could lead in serious cases to amputation (Anderson 2011, 24).

There were some moves towards compensation, support and rehabilitation for workers disabled through their work. Disablement and consequent incapacity of a breadwinner could plunge whole families into immediate poverty. The National Insurance Act of 1911 enabled workers to insure themselves against unemployment caused by accidents. Insured workers could in theory, under this law, be paid 30 shillings a week and receive health care and access to a doctor after an accident. However, these schemes were temporary and did not provide for long-term disablement, with benefits starting to reduce after 26 weeks. The Mining Industry Act of 1920 included some provision for care and rehabilitation through special hospitals and medical services. The Delevingne Committee Report of 1939 recommended an organised fracture service, to prevent disability arising from badly treated fractures, limb-fitting services for injured workers (equivalent to those in place for disabled ex-servicemen) and curative workshops in hospitals (Anderson 2011, 23–5).

As well as state and charitable support, for some disabled civilian workers (and their families) the burgeoning labour movement began to offer a third arena of support. Friendly society schemes in heavy industries with high rates of disablement, such as coalmining, had operated since the late 18th century, offering benefits and support to those unable to work because of illness or injury, and funded by small weekly contributions from workers (Turner and Blackie 2018). These, however, were primarily focused on providing support for temporary absence from work, and were less effective at meeting the needs of those permanently disabled and unable to return to their original jobs. From the late 19th century, working-class self-help in the form of special funds played an increasingly important role, certainly in heavy industry, in meeting the needs of disabled workers. After the First World War, trade unions became increasingly influential in establishing such funds. They would pay for items such as artificial limbs, wheelchairs and other specialist mobility equipment, artificial eyes and hearing amplifiers, as well as supporting rehabilitation and, where possible, some form of reintegration into the workforce (Curtis and Thompson 2014).

Despite these initiatives there was no over-riding structure of support in place for the physically disabled civilian, in contrast, as we shall see, to the more impressive system of support that was put in place for disabled ex-servicemen after the First World War. Disability, whether present from birth or acquired in childhood and adulthood, was, for any person without independent means, often a passport to lifelong deprivation. The situation was well set out by the *National Cripples' Journal*, first published in 1930, written by disabled people themselves and sold door to door:

> We want to get national recognition for crippled people in the same way as is given to the blind, our comrades in distress. We do not want to be dependent on charity, but want National Workshops with a living wage for partially disabled cripples, and for the poor cripple in the spinal carriage we want a small weekly pension instead of poor relief. It is dreadful to be totally disabled and also in distress.
>
> (quoted in Anderson 2011, 26–7)

War and its impact on disability

In November 1918, ten days before the armistice that would bring the First World War to an end, Clifford Allen wrote in his diary about a young woman and a discharged soldier living in a cottage near him in Surrey. 'He has lost both legs and propels himself about cheerfully in a mechanical chair. The other evening he was sitting talking to his bride when the kettle started to boil over. He forgot he had no legs and jumped up to seize the kettle only to fall into space on his sore stumps' (Gilbert 1995, 541). The young man was one of many tens of thousands who were having to become accustomed to a new and unfamiliar life as a disabled person.

The human toll of the First World War was appalling. Not only had almost one million British servicemen been killed, but almost two million had been wounded. In many cases their wounds caused permanent disabilities – amputated limbs, blindness, deafness and impaired mobility. There were mental as well as physical wounds. At the beginning of 1922 as many as 50,000 British soldiers were receiving government pensions for the ongoing impact of shell-shock on their minds (Gilbert 1995, 542).

The challenge to society was immense. There was an impact on a whole range of disability issues: rehabilitation, housing, employment, prosthetics, rights, and entitlement to assistance and support. Communities, policy makers and arms of local and national government struggled to absorb this influx of newly disabled men. There was also a challenge to eugenicist views. This was not disability that could be fallaciously explained away as the consequence of fecklessness or

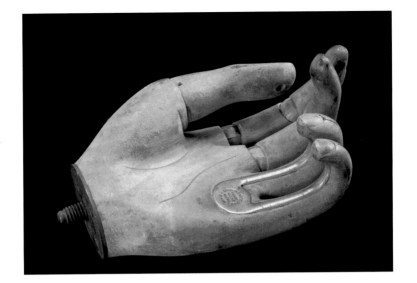

Fig 6.4
The First World War prompted rapid progress in the development of prosthetics – artificial left hand, Birmingham, 1920.
[Science Museum, London. Attribution 4.0 International (CC by 4.0)]

excessive breeding. It was disability arising from the willingness of these men, many of them from the very lower orders the eugenicists despised so much, to sacrifice their bodies and their minds in carrying out their patriotic duty to their country. There was a sense of obligation, that those who had sacrificed themselves should be paid back by society in the form of adequate support and assistance. They were the 'deserving' disabled, and tensions emerged between the idea of the deserving war disabled and the less-regarded civilian disabled.

New skills were acquired in response to this sudden exponential growth in disability prevalence. Queen Mary's hospital in Roehampton, London, became in 1915 the main English limb-fitting hospital for ex-servicemen. More than 40,000 lost one or more limbs during the conflict.

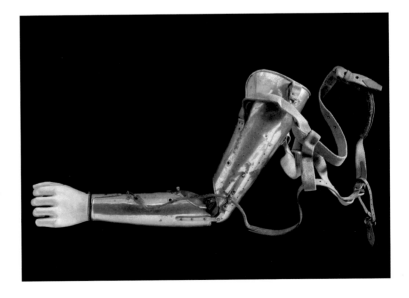

Fig 6.5
Artificial left arm, London, 1927.
[Science Museum, London. Attribution 4.0 International (CC by 4.0)]

Swamped by demand, the number of beds increased throughout the war. Limbs were made and fitted at Roehampton, then the recipients were trained in their use. There was an employment bureau at the hospital which helped amputees to find work. The Disabled Society, a war charity, agitated for lighter artificial limbs: light aluminium replaced heavy wooden legs and arms (Anderson 2011, 45) (Figs 6.4 and 6.5).

Many soldiers had been severely disfigured by gunshot wounds and shrapnel. Queen's Hospital in Sidcup, Kent, was a centre for facial surgery where the pioneering plastic surgeon Sir Harold Gillies developed maxillofacial surgery which reconstructed disfigured faces. The artist Francis Derwent-Wood worked there and applied his skills with burned patients to make masks concealing areas that surgery could not restore (Anderson 2011, 44).

Rehabilitation through exercise and sport became important. At the Croydon Union Workhouse Infirmary (later the Mayday Hospital) in Surrey, Colonel Deane established his gymnastic exercise centre for rehabilitation of disabled ex-servicemen. At St Dunstan's, a large property in 15 acres of Regent's Park, central London, 1,833 blinded ex-servicemen passed through, recuperating, learning skills and exercising. Members were taught Braille, typing, telephony, poultry keeping, vegetable gardening and basket making to prepare them for life when they returned

Fig 6.6

A band of seven blinded veterans play the banjo at St Dunstan's in London, 1918. [Wellcome Collection]

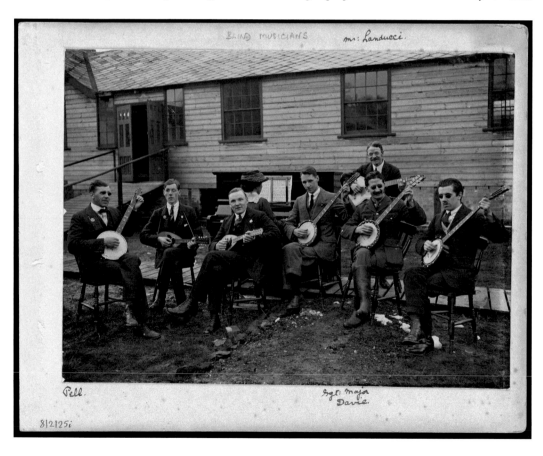

home, the aim being to retrain these blinded men in useful trades, or as *The Times* newspaper put it, 'to assist its men to become useful and productive citizens rather than idle and unhappy pensioners'. Their future happiness would be assured by their ability to contribute in some way. St Dunstan's and the men who lived there became a symbol of disabled heroism, regularly featured in the British press both during and after the war. A grateful public visited and 'made a fuss' of the men, accompanying them to theatres and concerts. Not all of St Dunstan's residents were impressed, and some expressed scepticism at the motives for the attention they were receiving and its likely longevity: 'Now we're the "fashion"; we're "those dear brave lads who've sacrificed so much" … but how long will it last?' (Anderson 2011, 49–53) (Fig 6.6).

The Star and Garter home for disabled soldiers and sailors opened in 1916 in Richmond, Surrey, with a sister home in Sandgate on the Kent coast. Rehabilitative work training included a poultry farm known as No-Man's Land. Agricultural work was seen as beneficial for men disabled and traumatised by war. There was even a pigeon loft, and the men participated in pigeon racing competitions. The home was predicated on a restoration of excitement, conviviality and a sense of independence to the lives of the young disabled veterans who lived there. A group of them travelled around driving specially constructed motorised Argson tricycles which could reach speeds of up to 15 miles per hour. On one occasion they went together to the Ascot races. They became known as the 'flying squad'. Their activities conveyed a sense both of their eagerness to regain their independence, and a longing for their former lives (Anderson 2011, 53–5).

Work and housing were particular concerns. The 'King's National Roll' was a 1919 scheme encouraging firms to employ disabled ex-servicemen, but its success rate was low. In 1927 a training school for war-disabled taxi drivers was set up in London. However, for the most part, disabled people, even the widely admired ex-soldiers, remained on the margins of economic activity. Most work opportunities were

Fig 6.7
A box containing poppies made by severely disabled ex-servicemen at the original British Legion poppy factory in King's Cross, London. [Collection of Auckland Museum]

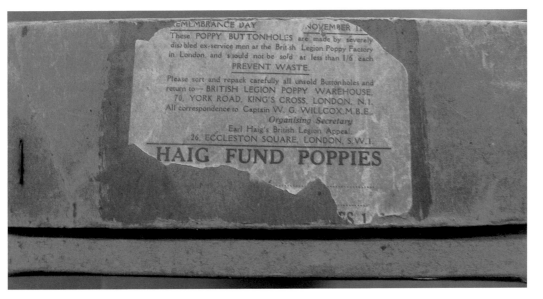

sheltered. Disabled men trained as limb fitters at Roehampton. The British
Legion opened its poppy factory in Richmond, Surrey (Fig 6.7).

A network of ex-servicemen's villages were built, providing sheltered
employment as well as family housing. These included Haig Homes in
Welwyn Garden City, Westfield War Memorial Village in Lancaster and
the Enham Village Settlement near Andover in Hampshire. There was also
specialist housing. In 1920, 12 cottages were funded from public donation
in Sprowston, near Norwich, for disabled members of the Royal Norfolk
Regiment. In 1927 the Prince of Wales opened the North Memorial
Homes in Leicester, 35 homes for disabled ex-servicemen.

There was thus a rapid adaptation by society to the needs of its large
newly-disabled population, built on a sense of obligation and reciprocity
for the sacrifices they had made. It was far from perfect and much of it
was charitable rather than state provided, and many disabled veterans
felt aggrieved at a lack of support. Nevertheless, it was a qualitatively
different response to that which most of the civilian disabled population
had experienced in the first half of the 20th century, and there was a clear
dichotomy between the two.

Some of the developments for ex-servicemen also benefited the
civilian disabled population. The new artificial limbs became available
to more civilians, specialist medical facilities for disabled miners were
introduced in the 1920s, and rehabilitation for industrial injuries was
considered in the 1930s. Many felt, however, that resources were not
evenly shared (although in fact pensions for disabled servicemen were
limited and their unemployment levels remained high). The British
Legion, a veterans' association, openly advocated preferential treatment
for veterans, arguing that in 'the making of provision for the handicapped
and their rehabilitation, the veterans come first'. Provision and support
for disabled civilians and children would have to come, they suggested,
from 'the more or less generous mercy of private or semi-private charity'.
At a 1920 conference on care of 'crippled' children, it was claimed that
provision for the war disabled had caused 'an appalling amount of
suffering' among other disabled people (Anderson 2011, 48–9).

The right to education – the growth of the 'special' school for disabled children

An Education Act of 1870, coming just three years after the franchise had
been extended to the urban working classes, required education provision
to be established for all 5–12-year-olds. Schooling then became obligatory
for all 5–10-year-olds in England and Wales in 1880. This universalisation
of education brought a spotlight, sometimes unwelcome and not always
sympathetic, onto the issue of schooling for disabled children. For the
most part, previously they had either been ignored or seen as having
a 'reasonable excuse' not to attend school. Now they became seen as a
'problem' by many educationalists.

As a result, the early 20th century, building on a raft of legislation in
the 1890s, saw a significant shift towards specialist education for disabled
children. The 1893 Elementary Education (Blind and Deaf Children)
Act shifted responsibility for education of deaf and blind children from

Poor Law authorities to local education authorities, who became obliged either to develop their own schools or support voluntary-sector provision. This Act was based on the findings of a Royal Commission which had recommended schooling for deaf and blind children to prevent them becoming not only 'a burden to themselves but a weighty burden to the state' (Borsay 2005, 106).

An Elementary Education (Defective and Epileptic Children) Act in 1899 empowered (but did not mandate) local authorities to provide schools for intellectually impaired children, or at least those of them deemed educable. The 1918 Education Act made schooling for all mentally and physically 'defective' children mandatory, although this was not implemented until the mid-1920s. It built on the 1893 Act, which had signalled a shift to local authority responsibility for schooling for blind and deaf children (Borsay 2005, 106–7).

There was, therefore, a welcome expansion of educational provision to children with disabilities, but much of it was specialist and therefore in consequence separated them from their non-disabled peers. It was often thought better for children to be away from their families, so for many the experience of education was residential, which meant that they also became separated from their own families and neighbourhoods. A small number of children attended mainstream schools, but the majority of provision was specialist. By the 1920s Britain had more than 500 institutions for children with sensory or physical impairments, of which around a quarter were for deaf or blind pupils (Borsay 2005, 108).

The voluntary education sector thrived, commissioned by local education authorities to take children for whom they were now obliged to secure an education. The Royal National Institute for the Blind (RNIB) set up a network of 'Sunshine Homes', which pioneered liberal and progressive teaching and care methods. The first was in Chorleywood, Hertfordshire, in 1918, and had an intake of 25 blind infants. The Chailey Heritage Craft School in Sussex was founded in 1903 under the banner of the 'Guild of the Brave Poor Things', the disabled group we encountered in Chapter 5. The school offered disabled children from deprived city areas craft training in a countryside setting, with the aim of ensuring independence in adulthood. Its powerful founder Grace Kimmins, steeped in the thinking of her time, called Chailey 'the public school of crippledom', whose aim was to 'remake' the disabled child through vocational training, education, recreation and medical care (Borsay 2005, 108).

There was often a focus on low-skilled work training rather than full education, and many educational regimes could be harsh and highly disciplinarian. Parental visits were discouraged and letters home censored. A group of blind boys made a night-time 'escape' from the Mount School for the Deaf and Blind in Stoke-on-Trent in 1915 because they wished to contribute to the war effort by working on a farm. When they returned they were placed with the deaf children as a punishment (because it would be difficult for them to communicate) and were forced to hand in their trousers each night to prevent further escapes (Humphries and Gordon 1992, 95–6) (Fig 6.8).

Such harshness meant that relations between staff and pupils were often combative. Pupils at the Manchester Road School for the Blind in Sheffield

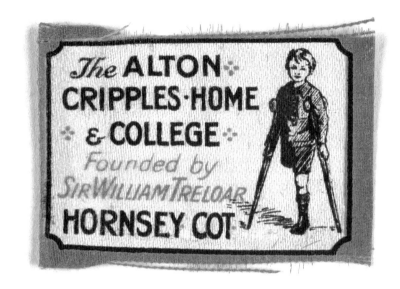

Fig 6.8
A charity flag for a boarding
school for disabled children,
1920s.
[Wellcome Collection]

went on a two-day strike in 1929 after a pupil was severely disciplined for
something he had not done. As one of them, Ted Williams, recalled:

> There was once a really popular boy in our class, Arthur Hayes, a grand
> personality. One of the teachers punished him for something he said and
> us boys all knew that he had not done. And, well, the teacher accused and
> punished him but all us boys, his friends and mates, stood by him. We
> organised a strike. We just refused to work in class. We sat there with our
> arms folded and wouldn't lift a finger … Even in the music class we just
> refused to sing. Of course we all got punished severely for striking and
> after a couple of days we were forced to give in to the teachers.
> (Humphries and Gordon 1992, 95)

Deaf children were often required to learn to lip read rather than use sign
language, which was usually their preferred method of communication.
There had been a long-standing dispute since the 1800s among deaf
educators, divided between 'oralists' who advocated teaching deaf
children to lip read and to learn to speak, and advocates of the signing
method, manualists, who saw signing as a language and a culturally
appropriate form of communication for deaf people. Oralists (usually not
themselves deaf) argued that lip reading and speaking allowed greater
integration into society, but also argued that signing was subversive
and dangerous, given that the majority of hearing people could not
understand what was being said (Safford and Safford 1996, 109–12).

This debate played out in schools for the deaf in the first half of
the 20th century. Sign language was normally banned in the classroom
because of this fear of subversion and secret communication. At the
Yorkshire Residential Institute for the Deaf in Doncaster pupils signed
with each other to maintain a secret, independent life, out of the sight of
staff. Joyce Nicholson recalled her time at the Birmingham Royal School
for the Deaf and Dumb in the 1920s:

> We were never allowed to sign in class at school. They tried to make us speak and to lipread which I really found difficult. We used to look forward to being out of the teacher's eye so we could sign. We used to sign behind their backs when they were writing on the blackboard with our hands under our desks. But if you were caught the teacher would be very angry. Sometimes we would get smacked on the hands and our arms would be tied by our sides … just to stop us from signing.

Hostility to signing, from hearing teachers, was intense, and the ironic effect was to make it the subversive, underground activity that the oralists feared (Humphries and Gordon 1992, 76–7, 84).

The sexes were rigorously separated, but boys and girls nevertheless found ways to communicate. Pupils from the Halliwick Home for Crippled Girls in Edmonton, North London, would slip crumpled notes to the choirboys on their weekly visits to church. In blind schools pupils would pass Braille love letters under the desk, with a punishment of caning and a lecture on wickedness if they were found out. In deaf schools signing would be used to arrange illicit meetings away from the gaze of punitive teachers. Eugenic panic fuelled the anxieties of teaching staff and school authorities about intermingling of male and female disabled pupils (Humphries and Gordon 1992, 106–8).

From Germany, the 'open-air school' came to England. Disabled children studied in a regime of outdoor classrooms, afternoon rest and improved diet. Even in winter they took afternoon naps outside wrapped in blankets. The first such school was opened by London County Council at Bostall Woods, Woolwich, in 1907. Away from unhealthy, crowded home environments, there would be, it was hoped, improvements in children's health. By 1939 there were 150 open-air schools, providing for almost 20,000 children (Anderson 2011, 20; Humphries and Gordon 1992, 60–2) (Fig 6.9).

The acquisition of the right to education was a great gain for children with disabilities, and special schools mushroomed across the country.

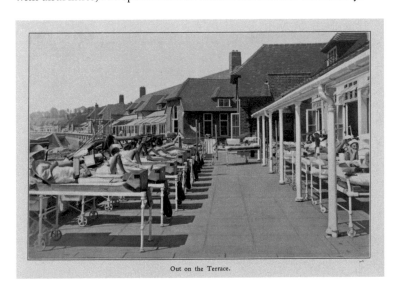

Out on the Terrace.

Fig 6.9
Open-air schools became popular between the wars – Lord Mayor Treloar's Cripples Hospital and College, Alton, Hampshire, 1937.
[Wellcome Collection]

Yet in practice it could prove a mixed blessing. For some it could be progressive and highly innovative. For others, it was a brutal and isolating experience. For most, it was the beginning of a life of separation.

'Mental deficiency' between the wars – life in the colony

In November 1917 as the First World War raged on, Leslie Scott, the chairman of the Central Association for the Care of the Mentally Defective, turned his mind to the looming problems of the peace. 'There are', he wrote, 'large numbers of low-grade, even imbecile defectives, now in remunerative work who will assuredly leave their work when there is any displacement of labour, and we are anxious to make plans for their protection'. Clearly, the country's need for manpower, with so many fighting on the front, had changed almost overnight the perception of the 'mentally deficient', from people incapable of work to useful members of the workforce (The National Archives, NATS 1/727). However, this was about to change again, as soldiers returned from the front with an expectation of employment.

There was a great irony to this communication. Those formerly known as idiots, and now repackaged as the mentally deficient by the medical profession who had decided that their care and 'treatment' was a medical duty, were the most viciously targeted by the eugenicists. A draconian Mental Deficiency Act has been passed with overwhelming cross-parliamentary support in 1913, after extensive pressure from the eugenicist lobby. The Act characterised the mentally deficient as incapable, dangerous, non-productive, a burden, and a threat to the health of the nation. The legislation sought their eventual eradication by preventing their capacity to reproduce, through a combined system of permanent institutionalisation and close community surveillance.

The Act's implementation, however, was put on hold by the outbreak of war. During the war many thousands of mentally deficient people, who had been deemed a parasitical drain on society in 1913, took up valuable and skilled work roles from 1914 to fill labour shortages caused by men departing for the front. As patients were discharged from mental hospitals to make way for wounded soldiers in need of treatment, some even joined the armed forces and fought at the front. It was a dramatic and rapid transformation from useless to useful, a stunning example of how social attitudes, circumstances and assumptions can construct the meaning of disability at any given time (Jarrett 2020, 267).

Their efforts were all to no avail in the long term. As war came to an end there was no reconsideration of the position of the mentally deficient in society. As society attempted to return to some form of normality and soldiers returned to civilian life from the front, their own peculiar normality returned for the mentally deficient: confinement to institutions and ostracisation from society. They were ejected from the factories and other workplaces where they had made their contribution, and a new era of intensive targeting of the so-called deficient began.

The 1913 Act had set up a new government Board of Control and specified that 'mental defectives' should either be closely supervised in the community or maintained in 'mental deficiency colonies', providing permanent settlement for both children and adults in an isolated 'scattered village' environment. These ideas of separation and control derived from the eugenic obsession with 'breeding'. It was argued that 'defective' members of the population would cause a general deterioration of the racial stock unless kept strictly controlled, segregated and, if possible, sterilised. Mental defectives were graded in the Act as follows:

a   Idiots: that is to say, persons so deeply defective in mind from birth or from an early age as to be unable to guard themselves against common physical dangers.

b   Imbeciles: that is to say, persons in whose case there exists from birth or from an early age mental defectiveness not amounting to idiocy, yet so pronounced that they are incapable of managing themselves or their affairs, or, in the case of children, being taught to do so.

c   Feeble minded persons: that is to say persons in whose case there exists from birth or an early age mental defectiveness not amounting to imbecility, yet so pronounced that they require care, supervision and control for their own protection, or for the protection of others, or, in the case of children, that they by reason of such defectiveness appear to be permanently incapable of receiving proper benefit from the instruction in schools.

d   Moral imbeciles: that is to say persons who from an early stage display some permanent mental defect coupled with strong vicious or criminal propensities on which punishment has had little or no deterrent effect.

These categorisations effectively divided people into two types. Idiots and imbeciles were helpless, and therefore useless, vulnerable and a burden. The feeble-minded and moral imbeciles had semi-developed minds and were therefore threatening and dangerous, because they could take on the appearance of 'normality' but lacked any sense of morality, restraint or real understanding. The moral imbecile was seen as being particularly dangerous because, according to the medical profession, they had certain capabilities, could appear 'normal', but were incapable of distinguishing right from wrong.

To house as many members of the defective population as possible, new colonies were established across the country, added to the existing supply of imbecile asylums and other institutions. Each was a small, self-contained world. Between 900 and 1,500 people would live in the typical colony, in detached 'villas' housing up to 60 people, grouped around a central administrative block. This block always formed a barrier between male and female villas, as separation of the sexes was deemed essential, except in the case of the lowest grade 'idiots'. Children and adults lived separately, and there would also be a special villa for 'difficult cases' – those whose behaviours were regarded as needing control. The villas for 'idiots' and for 'difficult cases' would be as far from the hospital approaches as possible, to avoid offence to visitors. Villas housing the 'better class of working patients' were allowed to be furthest from the administrative block, with their own cooking and heating facilities. Patients slept in multiple rows with beds closely stacked together in large dormitories. There was no space for privacy. For the lucky ones, there

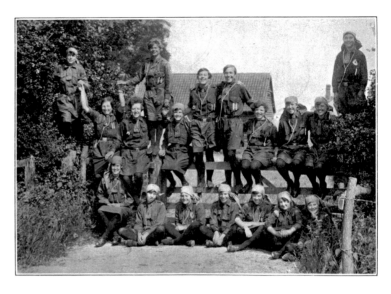

were small 'lockers' for the storage of their meagre personal possessions.

As well as the villas there would be a children's school, workshops for the adults, kitchens, bakery, laundry, recreation hall (seating up to 750 patients and doubling as a chapel), staff quarters, playing fields (particularly for the males) and a small mortuary. No one need ever leave. Many colonies had their own farms with market gardens, stables, poultry, pigs, herds of cows and greenhouses. As well as nurses, they employed farm bailiffs, firemen, engineers and, of course, gatekeepers. Most patients worked (unpaid) in the laundries and workshops or on the farm. The 'idiots' stayed in their villas, but these had verandas, so that they could be out in the fresh air even in bad weather. The children attended school, where they would learn useful occupational skills, but only for their future life as an adult in the colony (Jarrett 2020, 269–72) (Fig 6.10).

Outside the colonies, systems of guardianship and statutory or voluntary supervision were in place. Under guardianship, defectives living in their own homes were subject to the control of a suitable guardian, who could be a parent, other relative or employer. Under the supervision system, they were overseen through visits to their homes (often their family homes shared with their parents) by salaried officials, health visitors, school nurses, social workers or an overwhelmingly middle-class army of visitors from the Central Association for Mental Welfare, a voluntary body. The overriding aim of both the institutional and community systems was to prevent mixing and breeding. The mentally deficient had become the most surveilled, restricted and persecuted social group in the whole of Britain, perceived as a demonised biological fifth column in the body politic (Jarrett 2020, 271).

In 1939 another war came, and some 'colonists' left to work, or even fight. But the colonies would live on until the 1990s, renamed as mental handicap hospitals but not reformed.

Everyday life and work – disabled people in the community in the early 20th century

Although the number of disabled people in institutions grew markedly in the first half of the 20th century, the majority as ever still remained in their communities. However, it was a difficult time, with growing governmental supervision based on a fear of the spread of 'feeblemindedness' and degeneration. This was associated with people with physical, mental and sensory disabilities, as all were seen as somehow defective and deficient and therefore not belonging to the mainstream of society.

Those subjected to the home supervisory and monitoring visits of the middle-class watchdogs of the Central Association for Mental Welfare on behalf of the government's Board of Control, had strong memories of their 'benefactors'. These reveal the sheer scale of state intrusion into the lives of disabled people, supposedly living freely in their communities. One woman recalled the visiting Mr Grey. 'Grey! … Ooh I hated him! He wouldn't let anybody live. He did a lot of damage, picking up people what didn't deserve to be picked up.' Enthusiastic local branches of the Central Association identified large numbers of 'deficient people' for supervision. There were more than a thousand people under supervision or guardianship in the county of Somerset by 1929. Reports often carried a strong moral undertone, commenting for example on the cleanliness of the home. There was also a specific question to be answered by all health or volunteer visitors to 'a defective's home' on the risks of procreation: 'Is it considered that the control available would suffice to prevent the defective from procreating children?' An example of a positive answer to this query was 'Patient always in the care of either grandfather or mother.'

Reports could be positive: 'in spite of the girl's paralysis it is wonderful the amount of tasks she can perform in the house and she helps her grandmother all she can'. They could also be less than glowing: 'The home is a poor one, although there does not appear to be a lack of money.' Either way there was always the sense of a household with a 'defective' member needing to prove itself as morally acceptable and practically competent to prevent a move from supervision to institutionalisation, under the judgemental gaze of its middle-class visitors (Atkinson *et al* 1997 41, 119, 100–1).

The will to prevent sexual relationships and marriage was intense. In Rotherham in 1926, Mabel Miles, a 27-year-old 'defective' and her boyfriend Thomas Lancaster, a coal miner, applied for a marriage license. Mabel Miles's mother was opposed. 'No certificate is to be issued,' ruled the Board of Control, on the grounds that Miles had been detained in an institution between 1916 and 1926. The control of the state over people seen as having disabled minds stretched far beyond the institution (The National Archives 1926, RG48/159).

Because physical disability and sensory impairment were so rife, particularly among working-class children, in this period compulsory physical examinations were carried out in schools from 1907. It is likely that rather than there being an actual sudden increase in numbers, the introduction of such examinations had made the extent of disability clear, which may have simply gone unrecorded previously. Between the 1900s and 1950s an estimated half a million boys and girls had disabilities, often caused by diseases such as rickets, polio and TB, alongside the toll taken by high levels of road accidents in poor areas. The problems of poverty – poor housing, sanitation, health care and diet – allied with a lack of immunisation, were taking an immense toll (Anderson 2011, 17–18).

Loneliness, teasing and bullying could be a feature of daily life. 'I had no friends in the village. I used to go around more on a level with the dogs because I had to cross my legs over … and use them like a shovel to get about,' recalled Bob Hendley, who had polio as a young child in the 1920s. There were so-called 'cripple parlours', well-intentioned clubs for disabled children, but they could attract the derision of non-disabled children:

> It wasn't bad I suppose but you could only sit there, quite boring, and play dominoes or cards, maybe have a chat. As if that was the only place I was fit for and couldn't have had any fun anywhere else. I used to hate going in there if people were looking because of them shouting out names to you or laughing at you for going to a place with a name like that.

Others had happier memories of support and solidarity from family and friends. Gerald Turner, born in Rotherham in 1931, was fiercely and effectively defended by his siblings:

> There would be real fisticuffs, especially from my sister if ever someone started to make fun of me. My brothers and her stuck by me in our village when I were little. They used to take me out and play games so I could join in … You didn't have proper wheelchairs then. In the evenings quite often one of my brothers would get me on his back and we would all go off to the cinema to see a picture.

Gladys Berry who was born in Sheffield in 1912 with hereditary rickets, recalled being surrounded by good non-disabled friends:

> I could not walk at all, only shuffle on my bottom … and I was in a spinal carriage flat on my back for ages. I had some friends in our street and they treated me all right. In fact my best friends used to argue over who'd wheel me to the park, and when they were skipping in the street they used to let me turn one end of the skipping rope for them. I had a best friend, Hannah, and it was her that learnt me to walk when I was ten and started school.
>
> (Humphries and Gordon 1992, 39–41, 44–5)

Despite the mixed experiences of community life, there was always a strong link between disability and hardship. As we have seen, disabled people invariably found themselves at the bottom of the pile for employment, and any benefits they were able to receive were little above subsistence level. Some protested about their status and treatment. In 1920 and 1933, blind workers marched to London from all over Britain to hold mass demonstrations against low wages and poor working conditions. A culture of low expectations in schools for deaf, blind and 'crippled' children led many into low-skilled, repetitive jobs in sheltered workshops, if they were able to get any employment at all (Anderson 2011, 28–9).

Once again war changed everything. In 1941 the Ministry of Labour, faced with acute shortages, recruited more than 300,000 previously 'unemployable' disabled people into the workforce. 'Cripples Can Do Vital War Work' read a Northumbrian woman with cerebral palsy in a newspaper headline. Within months she was working at a Royal Ordnance Factory. 'It was a wonderful feeling … It was another step forwards … I revelled in being my own mistress at last' (Humphries and Gordon 1992, 133).

Yet again, people told in peacetime that they were incapable of work and did not belong in the workplace found themselves doing vital and skilled work when the demands of war called. There was no better illustration of the relative and shifting meaning of disability in society. In the same lifetime, and in the same society, one person could rapidly move from a perception that they were incapable of work and a burden to the community, to being perceived as a heroic, vitally included and contributing member. There was no stable meaning of what it meant to be disabled.

Mental illness, psychiatry and psychoanalysis

By the beginning of the 20th century medicine had staked its claim firmly on the terrain of the mind. Practitioners of the relatively new profession of psychiatry, which had developed over the 19th century, saw themselves very much as professional doctors of the mind and distanced themselves from the amateurish, eccentric mad doctors, quacks and faith healers that had preceded them. Their claim to exclusive understanding, diagnosis, treatment and control of madness led to some advances and innovations in treatment. It also led to much misery, exclusion and sometimes cruelty as the mentally ill became the object of their theories, experiments and custody.

A significant minority of those diagnosed as mentally ill continued to languish in long-stay hospital settings, the 19th-century asylum system still robustly in place as the new century began. Such systems of care were now tainted with the libel of eugenic science, seeing those whose minds were deranged or different as products of degeneration, immorality or weakness. Embedded in this viewpoint was the claim by the psychiatrists that mental illness was a disease, a scientific enterprise in which they could intervene and contribute alongside the biomedical sciences that were tackling bodily diseases. Patients were seen as symptom carriers, pathologised beings whose illnesses could be solved once the germs that caused the symptoms could be identified.

The German psychiatrist Emil Kraepelin (1856–1926) led this scientific drive, examining thousands of asylum patients and forming classifications based on disease concepts (Fig 6.11). He divided madness into two overarching categories. The first was a deteriorating, permanent condition he called 'Dementia Praecox', the second a more hopeful classification of manic-depressive psychosis, which could go

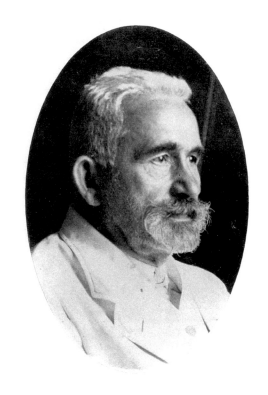

Fig 6.11

Emil Kraepelin.

[Wellcome Collection]

into remission. The Swiss psychiatrist Eugen Blueler (1857–1939) developed Kraepelin's Dementia Praecox idea into what he called 'schizophrenia', literally a splitting of the mind, which condemned the patient to a life of mental disaster, disorder and failed social relationships (Scull 2015, 263; Porter 2002, 183–6).

These medical ideas and claims brought a sense of gloom and helplessness to the understanding of mental illness and, combined with eugenic fears of degeneration, pathologised and demonised those who were labelled as mentally ill. The new language of madness was harsh and alienating. A British psychiatrist complained that degenerates were born every year 'with pedigrees that would condemn puppies to [drowning in] the horsepond'. Psychiatrists appeared to have become little more than well-armed border guards, protecting society from those on the wrong side of the mind (Scull 2015, 265; Porter 2002, 186).

There was, however, a contrasting pathway taken by one faction of mind doctors. In the early 20th century Sigmund Freud announced his profoundly original analysis of mental disturbance with his theory that the repression of unconscious mental states, in particular infantile sexuality, brought neurotic consequences in later life (Fig 6.12). The key to unlocking these processes was the practice of psychoanalysis, which became popularly known as the talking cure, where a patient would unearth their mental conflicts in a dynamic interaction with their analyst, leading to the cure of their neuroses. Psychoanalysis was influential in Britain, its practice led by Freud's Welsh acolyte, biographer, and right-hand man Ernest Jones. The Tavistock Clinic in London opened in 1920 to provide a focus for psychoanalytic practice. Jones daringly flew into Vienna in 1938 after the Nazi invasion of Austria to organise the extraction of Freud and his family to London from the inevitable fate that would await him, as an eminent Jewish intellectual, at the hands of the Nazis. Freud, already terminally ill, lived out the last year of his life in a house in Hampstead, London, now the site of the Freud Museum. However, much of mainstream British psychiatry remained unremittingly hostile to the talking cure, dismissing morbid introspection and regarding unsettling memories as best left undisturbed (Scull 2015, 322–7; Porter 2002, 188–93).

The talking cure was, however, influential in the understanding and treatment of what became known as 'shell shock' (Fig 6.13). Thousands of soldiers who had witnessed the horrors of mutilation and slaughter, and experienced the traumas of continuous bombardment and lethal combat, exhibited symptoms such as muteness, blindness, paralysis, shaking, screaming and uncontrolled gait with no apparent physical cause. Army commanders saw these as faked, the deliberate actions of cowards seeking to avoid their fighting duties. Army psychiatrists began

INTRODUCTORY
LECTURES ON
PSYCHO-ANALYSIS

A COURSE OF TWENTY-EIGHT
LECTURES DELIVERED AT
THE UNIVERSITY OF VIENNA

BY

PROF. SIGM. FREUD, M.D., LL.D.
VIENNA

AUTHORIZED ENGLISH TRANSLATION
BY
JOAN RIVIERE

WITH A PREFACE
BY
ERNEST JONES, M.D.
President of the International Psycho-Analytical Association

LONDON: GEORGE ALLEN & UNWIN LTD.
RUSKIN HOUSE, 40 MUSEUM STREET, W.C. 1

Fig 6.12
Freud's psychoanalytic theory
revolutionised understanding
of the unconscious mind.
[Wellcome Collection]

to see it differently, a traumatised nervous system in the brain reacting physically to what it had endured. The Cambridge neurologist W H R Rivers used Freudian-influenced psychotherapeutic techniques to treat his patients, who included the war poets Siegfried Sassoon and Wilfred Owen. This work was influential in developing an understanding of what would later become known as post-traumatic stress disorder (PTSD) (Scull 2015, 295–7).

Psychiatry thus stood divided in the first half of the 20th century. Was mental illness a disease to be treated with seclusion and the same medical interventions, however invasive or brutal, that any physical disease might require? Or did it have wild, deep psychological roots, that the skilled therapist could encourage the patient to unearth from the depths of their unconscious, beneath the calm veneer of civilisation? Was mental illness something to be cut or coaxed from the human mind?

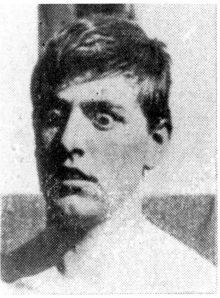

Fig 6.13
The 'talking cure' led to a more
sympathetic understanding
of shell shock (later post-
traumatic stress disorder).
[Wellcome Collection]

Conclusion

The early part of the 20th century was, on the whole, a miserable and stigmatising period for people with any type of disability. Prevalence of physical disability, blindness and deafness was high, fuelled by poverty, poor healthcare, disease and unhealthy, dangerous environments. A divide opened up between the 'deserving disabled' who had sacrificed their bodies in war, and the civilian disabled. There were advances in provision of education to children with disabilities, but separation into specialist educational settings, while successful at times, often created isolating and punitive environments and perpetuated lifelong pathways of separation and segregation. Nineteenth-century asylums lingered on as long-stay hospitals, bleak and, too often, cruel environments.

The eugenic libel identified people with mental or physical disabilities as a threat to health, a danger to the future of society unless action was taken. This was perhaps the worst period in history for the 'mentally deficient' – legislation sought to eradicate them altogether through institutionalisation, separation, surveillance and the prevention of procreation. A trend towards a disease model of mental illness meant that the mentally ill fared little better. As the world slipped once more into war in 1939, it was perhaps inevitable that the social war on disabled people that had characterised the preceding decades would evolve into something even more horrific.

Discussion: Models of disability

The 'medical model' played an increasingly important role in the lives of disabled people over this period. Why did medicine stake a claim to 'treat' disability, and was this claim fair? What is the 'social model of disability' and why are there such heated debates about these two competing models?

The 'medical model' of disability is defined as the domination of medical experts and medical treatments of disability. When the medical model is in operation, this plays out both in everyday social and cultural life and also in how disability history is understood. Medical practitioners are seen as the power group who have the right to identify, diagnose, treat and manage disability. Their job is to cure the disability, alleviate its impact or else to manage the lives of those with incurable disabilities, often in some sort of medical institution. They are seen as the holders of knowledge and authority, the disabled person playing very much a secondary role as the object of this authority.

When disability history is understood through the medical model, then it becomes the story of medical advances in countering, or dealing with, disability. Such histories might include medical breakthroughs such as vaccination against polio, which has been successful in eradicating a dangerous and highly contagious disabling disease, or successes in developing prosthetics or other technologies that improve the lives of disabled people. They will also recount the lives of great medical practitioners in the field of disability or disease, such as the physician Edward Jenner, who pioneered the use of vaccines in the 18th century,

John Langdon Down who identified what he called Mongolian Imbecility and which later became known as Down syndrome, or the neurosurgeon Ludwig Guttmann, whose work inspired what became the Paralympics.

While it is undoubtedly true that there have been inspirational members of the medical profession who have made significant contributions to improve the lives of disabled people, campaigners, activists and historians have identified a number of problems with the medical model. First, not all medical interventions in the world of disability have been progressive or benign – one need only look at the medically managed asylum system of the 19th century, the cruelties of 'corrective' surgery in the 20th, and the ongoing scandals of medicalised institutional care for people with mental illness and learning disabilities today to know that medical intervention does not always represent progress and improvement.

Second, the medical focus on disability tends to reinforce the assumption that disability is some sort of individual tragedy that needs to be eradicated or dealt with in some way. Disabled people are seen as a medical problem, and defined solely by their level of 'defect' against a normative standard of bodily functioning.

Finally, the voice of the disabled person is seen as secondary to the authority of medicine, and medicalised pathways of treatment are imposed without the person's involvement or sometimes even consent. They are therefore dehumanised and objectified to some extent, and their status as an individual, a social being, is neglected or ignored. In medicalised histories, individual stories of disabled people are buried beneath narratives of medical progress and triumphant medical practitioners.

From the 1960s, radical critics, many of them disabled themselves, challenged the medical model, and developed a new theory of disability known as the social model. They did not see disability as an individual issue, in which society needed to deal with the 'personal trouble' of those who deviated from the norm. Rather, they saw disability as a public issue and argued that the problems of disabled people were not caused so much by the impairments that they were born with or acquired, but rather by economic, social and political factors which left them discriminated against, in poverty and excluded from everyday life. Thus, they developed a radical distinction between 'impairment' and 'disability'. In 1979 the Union of the Physically Impaired Against Segregation (UPIAS) defined impairment as 'lacking all or part of a limb or having a defective limb, organ or mechanism of the body'. In contrast, they described disability as 'the disadvantage or restriction caused by a contemporary social organization which takes no or little account of people who have physical impairments and this excludes them from the mainstream of social activities' (Borsay 2005, 10).

In other words, the argument of the social model was that while people were born with impairments which were real enough, it was society and its institutions that disabled them. A lack of physical adaptation, discrimination in employment, poverty and embeddedness in the benefits system, poor education, an absence of aspiration, public hostility, bad housing and other social and political factors combined to exclude impaired people from society. It was this socially created exclusion that was the disability, not the absence of a limb or the absence of sight or hearing.

Just as society could create exclusion, it was argued that it could also break it down if only it had the political will to do so. In the same way, the word 'handicapped', which had been widely used to describe disabled people (they were 'the mentally or physically handicapped'), took on a new meaning. For advocates of the social model, a handicap was something imposed on people by society. A person was handicapped from entering a building, not by the impairment of having no legs, but by the handicap of the staircase that they could not climb in their wheelchair, and the absence of a ramp. Society imposed the handicap, it was not innate.

The left-wing disability theorists Michael Oliver and Colin Barnes summed it up as follows in 1998:

> In the past twenty years our understanding of disability has changed radically. We have gone from viewing 'disability' as a tragic problem occurring for isolated, unfortunate individuals for whom the only appropriate social response was medical treatment, to seeing it as a situation of collective institutional discrimination and social oppression to which the only appropriate response is political action. Somewhere in between sits the welfare state, based neither wholly on personal tragedy theory nor fully embracing social oppression theory.
>
> (Oliver and Barnes 1998, 3)

For Barnes and Oliver and other proponents of the social model, it is not the person with a disability that must change to adapt to the society they were born into, it is society that must adapt to include, and ensure equal treatment for, all its members (Fig 6.14).

The social model of disability has largely supplanted the medical model in recent decades, thanks to the campaigning work of disabled people and the acute analysis of disabled theorists such as Barnes, Oliver and many others. There has, however, more recently been some criticism of the social model itself, on the grounds that it is too 'binary', presenting disability as a straightforward opposition between an oppressive

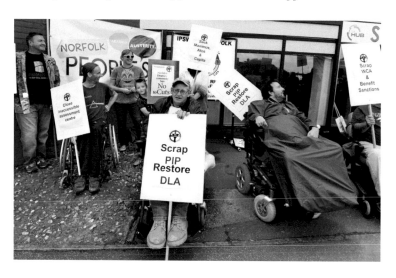

Fig 6.14
The social model of disability sees social oppression as the root cause of problems for disabled people.
[Roger Blackwell]

society and oppressed groups labelled as disabled. The model has also been criticised as too 'materialist', meaning that disability is explained exclusively in material, structural contexts such as economics and politics.

Such critics argue that disability should be understood more as a cultural matter, where the lived experience of the impaired person combines with a host of other factors, such as cultural assumptions and social interactions, language and attitudes as well as political, economic and social circumstances, to create the life experiences, positive and negative, of disabled people. They are particularly interested in the way medical conditions presented as unassailable scientific facts by medical practitioners can be loaded with meanings and assumptions that have little to do with science. The cultural model is itself critiqued by some activists and theorists for its excessive focus on language, symbols and meanings (or 'texts' as they are called by cultural theorists) rather than on the practicalities, biological realities and economic challenges that affect the lives of disabled people (Shakespeare 2014, 49–56).

The discussion of models of disability can sound rarefied and academic at times, removed from the concerns of everyday life. However, the prism through which disability is framed is a critical factor in how disabled people perceive themselves and are perceived by those among whom they live. This in turn is significantly instrumental in determining the everyday lives that people lead. Without the challenge of the social model, the excluding medical model would continue to shape common understandings of disability, and would manifest itself not only in books of theory but also in classrooms, workplaces, doctors' surgeries, hospitals, shops and all the other everyday settings that people encounter throughout their lives.

7 Out of the asylum, 1945–present

Introduction and summary

As the Second World War (1939–45) ended, the true extent of its horrors began to emerge. Among these was the mass killing of tens of thousands of disabled people in Germany in the name of racial and eugenic 'science'. Little appetite remained for the eugenicist theories that had circulated in the pre-war period advocating the isolation and sterilisation of disabled people. In England, a legacy of war was 300,000 newly disabled servicemen and women and civilians. The focus of public concern, as it had done after the First World War, shifted to the rehabilitation and support of those who had sacrificed their bodies for their country.

The Disability Employment Act of 1944 promised sheltered employment, reserved occupations and employment quotas for disabled people. Rehabilitation practices that had developed during the war, aimed at restoring the fitness, mobility, daily living skills and morale of disabled servicemen and women, spread to the civilian population. The new National Health Service took over and extended rehabilitation centres and services from 1948, including those aimed at workers disabled by industrial accidents.

Attitudes changed. Disabled people were not prepared to remain passive and, beginning with a 'silent reproach' march of disabled ex-servicemen in 1951, a social movement developed. A host of campaigning disability charity groups formed in the 1940s and 1950s. Through the 1960s and 1970s, inspired by the civil rights movement in America, direct action groups of disabled people campaigned against discrimination, poor access and inequality. In 1995 a Disability Discrimination Act was passed. The right to employment was often at the heart of these campaigns.

In this period disability campaigners and activists developed a clear focus on people's rights. How could disabled people be as much a part of society as everyone else? As well as rights to education and work, questions of physical access became critical. How could disabled people negotiate the complex environments of rapidly urbanising England without adjustments and adaptations being made? Dropped kerbs, accessible toilets and accessible buildings became key issues. At first there was a 'micro-approach', building separate specialist disabled facilities. This changed, and architects and planners began to embrace the ideas of 'universal design' – buildings and landscapes which enable every person to use every part of them.

Great changes took place in the arena of sport. Under the leadership of the inspirational refugee neurosurgeon Ludwig Guttmann, war-injured paralysed patients at Stoke Mandeville Hospital in Buckinghamshire began to compete against each other as part of their rehabilitation. In 1948 a wheelchair archery competition took place on the lawns of the hospital against other wheelchair users. It was the birth of the

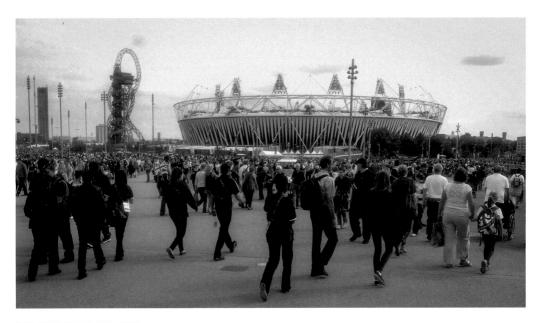

Fig 7.1
Crowds flock to the
Paralympics in the universal
design London Stadium, 2012.
[Gary Knight]

Paralympic Games (Fig 7.1). Today these games constitute a genuinely global sporting event, featuring elite disabled athletes who have become sporting icons in their own right.

Finally, the era of the asylum came to an end. Although they had lingered as long-stay hospitals after the war, a series of scandals revealed neglect and abuse, causing rising public concern. From 1981 the 'care in the community' programme signalled the end of the long-stay hospital, and tens of thousands of people with learning disabilities and mental health needs returned to life within mainstream communities. The Victorian ideal of safe institutional 'asylum' in rural settings, which had always lightly concealed an exclusionary mindset, ended as a shameful dystopian nightmare of containment, abuse and neglect. Today new hopeful visions of equality, inclusion and universal access have replaced it. Their long-term impact will be seen with time.

Disability and rehabilitation

The treatment of seriously injured, burned and disabled soldiers and civilians during the Second World War had been predicated on restoring them to participation in the war effort or, if that was not fully possible, to at least reduce dependence on assistance for the rest of their lives. Rehabilitation was all. An important element of the rehabilitative approach was that disability was no longer seen as necessarily an obstacle to employment at any level. The war effort required the return of injured and disabled members of the armed forces either to full duties or to some form of alternative duties as swiftly as possible. An iconic symbol of this philosophy was the pilot Douglas Bader, who was accepted as an RAF pilot during the war, despite having lost both legs in a flying accident in 1931.

New approaches brought new ideas in the concept of rehabilitation. Medical and surgical interventions to restore the body as fully as possible came to be seen as the first part of a process which then focused on restoration of fitness and mobility, relearning daily living skills and combating depression through purposeful activity, including work. The physiotherapy profession grew enormously. A 'Massage Corps' was established in 1938, and by 1942 it had 6,000 members supporting injured and disabled troops around the world. In 1943 it was renamed as the Physiotherapy Service. There were significant advances in the design and manufacture of artificial and prosthetic limbs, particularly at Roehampton Hospital, south London, which linked in to the wider rehabilitative process (Anderson 2011, 76–7, 180).

Rehabilitation became a fundamental component of the process for health intervention and support. It was also known by a number of other watchwords such as 'resettlement', 'reablement' and 'habilitation'. The Tomlinson Committee of 1943 embedded rehabilitation as a clinical practice, providing the basis for much of the rehabilitative and employment legislation adopted during and after the war. It described rehabilitation 'in its strictly medical sense [as] ... the process of preventing or restoring the loss of muscle tone, restoring the full functions of the limbs, and maintaining the patient's general health and strength'. It also acknowledged that rehabilitation was about the restoration of confidence, self-worth through occupation, the acquisition of skills to enable a return to work, and integration back into society wherever possible. During the medical treatment phase, early remedial techniques were introduced, such as bed exercise regimes, occupational therapy including basket making and rug weaving, repetitive exercises using legs and pullies and, later, sports and games. From hospital patients would move to a growing network of rehabilitation centres, such as Egham in Surrey, which operated as an experimental military centre from 1943. Such centres offered a programme of physical therapy, remedial gymnastics, sport and employment training (Anderson 2011, 75, 79, 80–1, 180–1).

One of the effects of the Tomlinson report was the application of rehabilitative approaches to civilian disabled people. After the war ended in 1945, the burgeoning collection of convalescent and rehabilitation centres for disabled servicemen and women that had grown up around the country started to open their doors to the wider population. In 1946 the Egham Centre, renamed the Egham Industrial Rehabilitation Centre, opened to civilians. It offered 'vocational guidance and purposeful training', particularly in building work, shoe repair and retail distribution. Roffey Park in Sussex specialised in supporting workers with mental health issues. St Dunstan's in Regent's Park, London, continued its rehabilitative work with blind servicemen, as did the RNIB with the rest of the blind population. The National Health Service had taken over most rehabilitation services by 1951, three years after its creation. Among these was the Miners' Rehabilitation Service, which included centres at Berry Hill Hall near Mansfield and the Hermitage in Chester le Street, Durham. In the 1960s the Daily Living Research Unit at Mary Marlborough Lodge, based at the Nuffield Orthopaedic Hospital in Oxford, pioneered new rehabilitative techniques in daily living skills and new designs in wheelchairs and appliances (Anderson 2011, 181–2).

Disability and work

Work was seen as crucial, both for rehabilitation purposes and to reduce dependence on the state in an era of labour shortages. The Disabled Persons (Employment) Act was introduced in 1944. This set out a programme of training and resettlement programmes, a scheme which required larger employers to recruit 3 per cent of their workforces from the cohort of registered disabled people, and segregated special workshops. Following this Act a group of factories was established – at first known as 'British Factories' and later renamed Remploy. The first of these was set up in Salford in 1946. By 1953 there were 90 such factories, employing 6,000 disabled people. Products included woodwork, leatherwork, mats and brushes. In Bristol and Halifax stump socks were manufactured for amputees. Veterans worked in the Thermega electric blanket factory in Ashtead, Surrey. Outside these sheltered work settings a registration scheme was set up requiring employers to take a fixed percentage of disabled workers. Certain occupations – lift operator and car park attendant – were reserved for disabled people.

The Disabled Persons (Employment) Act, although a welcome acknowledgement of and pragmatic response to the exclusion of disabled people from the labour market, was controversial in two ways. First, it embedded a division between 'normal' and 'abnormal' workers, marking a sharp differential between what were referred to as 'effective workers able to take their place in open employment' and 'ineffective workers for whom sheltered employment would be provided'. Second, it favoured those disabled in war over 'civilian' disabled. When the legislation was being drafted it was considered that there was little merit in discriminating between people disabled in battle and those born disabled or disabled in an industrial or civilian capacity. However, the parliamentarians Ian Fraser and Brunel Cohen advocated on behalf of veterans for them to be prioritised. Fraser had been blinded and Cohen had lost both legs when serving in the First World War, and saw themselves as the voice of the disabled veteran. As a result of their lobbying, the Act contained specialist schemes which offered veterans opportunities for higher education and access to grants to set up small businesses (Borsay 2005, 135; Anderson 2011, 183–4, 92–7).

Nevertheless, the Act was an important development in the recognition of the employment needs of disabled people and of the barriers they faced in employment. It was notable for recognising the employment needs of women with disabilities. In contrast to the First World War, there had been significant numbers of women casualties in the Second World War, both civilian and military. The Act specifically recognised the employment capacities and needs of disabled women. Some occupations for trainees were listed 'for women only', including parachute-making machinists. In 1948 a residential workshop for women with disabilities was established in Farnham in Surrey, where toys were made. The Ministry of Education collaborated with the Ministry of Labour in the Education Act of 1944 to provide vocational training for disabled children, juvenile employment officers to assist with pathways into employment, and vocational training centres for those school leavers unable to find work on leaving school. There were 67 of these centres by

1946, as well as industrial rehabilitation units for more severely disabled adults, specialising in light industrial work (Anderson 2011, 169, 193–4).

Despite these policy initiatives and state interventions, unemployment rates among disabled people remained high, as did the income gap between disabled people who were in work and the non-disabled workforce. Support available to those disabled by war remained at significantly higher levels than that available to the civilian disabled. Recognising these deeply embedded anomalies, and the strength of social belief in work as a necessary instrument of equality, the Disablement Income Group (DIG) was formed in 1965. This campaign group was founded by two disabled 'housewives', Megan du Boisson and Berit Moore, after they wrote a letter to *The Guardian* newspaper. Recognising that through the social security system people injured in war or the workplace were entitled to significantly more support than 'civilian' disabled, the group campaigned for a full disability income across all disability groups, regardless of the cause of their disability. The group was notable for having been founded by two women, and brought to public attention the injustice that disabled women were significantly disadvantaged by the focus on disability arising from war or workplace accidents. Their campaign, coupled with the thalidomide scandal of the 1960s, where a number of children with disabilities were born to women who had used the drug during pregnancy, led to the introduction of new social security benefits in the 1970s which did not discriminate against women who had never been in paid work. DIG was an early pioneer of the disability rights movement in the United Kingdom, its narrow focus on employment and benefit issues showing the central importance of issues around work and poverty in the lives of disabled people at the time.

Concerns about a culture of low expectations which encouraged segregation and the channelling of disabled people into low-skilled jobs brought about a move from sheltered work settings and a drive for inclusion in mainstream employment, in line with the idea of full participation in mainstream life. At the beginning of the 21st century, Remploy closed most of its factories and switched its focus to supporting disabled people into employment. Nevertheless, the move from segregated settings has not brought about a commensurate rise in employment rates for disabled people in the open market. Unemployment remains far higher than among the non-disabled population. High-profile disabled people such as the blind politician David Blunkett, who became the UK Home Secretary in 2001, the scientist Stephen Hawking and the athlete Tanni Grey-Thompson have reached the top of their professions. Yet unemployment, and poverty rates, among disabled people remain an issue, with a significant impact on any progression towards equality and inclusion.

Nowhere out of bounds – disability access and adaptation

From 1945 the pace of urbanisation of the English landscape quickened. With 300,000 war-disabled people added to the existing disabled population, issues of mobility and access in towns and cities became paramount. If the idea was that disabled people should work and participate in society, how could they do this amidst the complex buildings, difficult entrances and exits, steps, stairs, kerbs, busy roads and transport systems of the modern urban environment?

At this time the vast majority of buildings were not designed with disabled people in mind. A young architecture graduate, Selwyn Goldsmith (1932–2011), contracted poliomyelitis during a trip to Italy, disabling the right side of his body. This turned out to be a transformative event, and was instrumental in causing Goldsmith to devote the rest of his professional career to overcoming what he called 'architectural disability'. He fought the 'institutional discrimination' of buildings which placed impediments in the way of disabled people who wished to use them. Goldsmith was always careful to emphasise that the category of disability, in architectural terms, meant not just people using wheelchairs, but included also people who were deaf, blind people, the ambulant disabled and indeed anybody who had difficulty in negotiating buildings.

In 1961 Goldsmith was commissioned by the Royal Institute of British Architects (RIBA) to produce the first architectural guidance manual that focused on access to, and accessibility within, buildings. The result was his *Designing for the Disabled* (1963). This quickly became an indispensable 'bible' and teaching aid for architects and local authority planners who, until then, had paid little attention to accessibility issues.

In 1964 Goldsmith was commissioned as a 'research architect' to undertake a study of accessibility, specifically focused on people who used wheelchairs in Norwich in the east of England, which was selected as a representative English city. He relocated with his family and lived there for three years, working with Norwich Corporation. He interviewed 284 disabled people, asking which types of buildings should be made easier for disabled people to use. The highest priority by far was public toilets. The other buildings mentioned – restaurants, local shops, churches – reflected the desire of disabled people simply to lead the ordinary lives that other people led. From this came England's first unisex, disabled-access public toilet (on Castle Hill in Norwich) and Goldsmith's invention of the ramped, or dropped, kerb. Fifteen of them were established around the city, and they have now become a standard feature of urban design around the world.

The work in Norwich also produced the *Norwich Guide Book for Disabled People* and led to a revised edition of *Designing for the Disabled* in 1967. New knowledge about accessibility was evolving fast, much of it driven by Goldsmith's highly focused work. New accessible design innovations increasingly became a feature of English towns and cities. The fulfilment of Goldsmith's desire that all disabilities should be considered in such features can be seen in the example of the pelican (pedestrian light controlled) crossing, introduced in the UK in 1969. Dropped kerbs allow wheelchair users and people with mobility problems to cross easily, high-pitched bleeping, vibrating buttons or tactile rotating cones indicate to blind people that it is safe to cross, and lowered buttons enable wheelchair users to initiate the process of halting traffic (McIntyre 2015; Goldsmith 1963) (Figs 7.2 and 7.3).

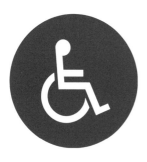

Fig 7.2
The wheelchair accessible
logo has become a common
sight in towns and cities.
[Manjiro5]

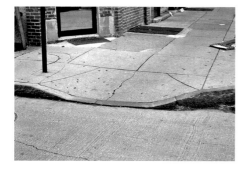

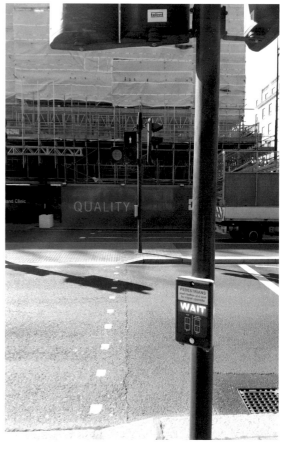

Fig 7.3
Pelican crossings have a number of accessibility
features.
[Plnms]

Fig 7.4
A wheelchair user in front of a block of accessibly
designed low-rise flats in Islington, London, in
1977.
[© Historic England Archive AA066616]

In 1970 the Chronically Sick and Disabled Persons Act required local authorities to have regard to disabled people when framing housing policies, and to help with arranging adaptation work to existing properties. Under the 1974 Housing Act, disabled people were able to apply for discretionary home improvement grants including the replacement of basic amenities such as baths and toilets if existing facilities were inaccessible due to people's impairment. In 1974 it was recognised that adaptation was not only important for wheelchair users but also for the ambulant disabled, and that there needed to be two concepts of special housing to accommodate the needs of these differing groups. In 1976 The Chronically Sick and Disabled Persons Act added workplaces to the list of premises that were required to be made accessible (Borsay 2005, 174, 281) (Fig 7.4).

Despite the improvements and innovations introduced as a result of Goldsmith's work and the raft of 1970s legislation, problems of physical access continued to present significant obstacles to disabled people. This was a major factor in ongoing exclusion from public life, employment and everyday activities such as travel on public transport, eating in cafes or restaurants, shopping and entertainment. Disabled people took the fight to the streets. In the 1990s Direct Action Network (DAN) and other organisations demonstrated against inaccessible public transport and buildings. On one occasion they blocked Westminster Bridge in central London, next to Parliament, lying in front of, and in some cases chaining themselves to, buses. One of the demonstrators, Jane Campbell, chair of the British Council of Disabled People (BCODP), described the discomfort of police officers dealing with disabled, wheelchair-using activists for the first time: 'They didn't know whether to arrest us or pat us on the head and give us an ice cream' (Kelly 2021).

In response to these pressures, government regulation consistently increased the onus on building owners to ensure that all public buildings were accessible and contained suitable facilities. This culminated in the Disability Discrimination Act (1995), which placed a duty on owners to take measures to make buildings accessible. The Act made it illegal to discriminate against disabled people 'in connection with employment, the provision of goods, facilities and services or the disposal or management of premises'. In each of these areas accessibility became a legal obligation – failure to allow access became, in theory at least, a punishable offence.

What Goldsmith described as a 'doctrinal leap' then took place, moving away from adding special facilities to a 'normal' building to the concept of 'universal design'. This saw any person with any disability as entitled to use every part of a building rather than having specialist additions within the building such as disabled-access toilets, while other toilets remained inaccessible. This was outlined in his 1997 text *Designing for the Disabled: A New Paradigm*. The idea of universal design was that not only should disabled people have physical access to every part of a building, but so should anyone else who might experience obstacles to getting around: parents with prams, people carrying heavy loads, elderly people and small children. As Goldsmith put it:

> The architect who takes the bottom-up route to universal design works
> on the premise that the building users he or she is serving, including

those with disabilities, are all people who can be treated as normal people. The architect does not start with the presumption that disabled people are abnormal, are peculiar and different, and that, in order to make buildings accessible to them, they should be packaged together and then, with a set of special-for-the-disabled accessibility standards, have their requirements presented in top-down mode as add-ons to unspecified normal provision.

He added 'I wish when I use buildings to do so in the same way as others, to be integrated rather than segregated, to be treated as a normal and not as a peculiar person' (Goldsmith, 1997).

The Richard Attenborough Centre for Disability and the Arts in Leicester provides an example of a complex but accessible multistorey public space. Architectural competitions now include accessibility as a key component for any award. The winner of the 2011 Stirling Prize, awarded by the RIBA for the UK's best new building, was the Evelyn Grace Academy in south London, a multilevel mainstream school on a cramped inner-city site – fully accessible throughout.

The impulse of much design is now not just about people being able to get into buildings, it is about them being able to get anywhere. In 2004 new design and landscaping features made the Tower of London, a thousand-year-old world heritage site, accessible. Some seaside resorts now have disabled access beach-huts. Nowhere should be out of bounds. Goldsmith's fight against 'architectural disability' lives on as, unfortunately, many access problems persist.

Disability and sport – the birth of the Paralympics, from rehabilitation to world-class performance

The disability sports movement began in earnest in 1944 with a competitive 'dressing exercise' on what was known as Ward X at Stoke Mandeville hospital, Buckinghamshire. The war-injured, paralysed young men on the ward raced each other to get up from their beds, dress and get into their wheelchairs.

Twelve spinal units had been set up around the country during the Second World War. However, it was Stoke Mandeville's director Ludwig Guttmann (1899–1980), a German Jewish neurosurgeon and refugee from Nazism, who made the first significant breakthrough in the rehabilitation of people with spinal paralysis through, among other interventions, the introduction of competitive sport (Fig 7.5).

Previously such people had been seen as 'hopeless cases'. At the beginning of the war the prognosis for servicemen paralysed by spinal injury was as bad as it had been in 1918. Mortality within the first few months of paralysis was as high as 65 per cent, usually following complications such as bed sores and urinary tract infections. The plaster beds used to transport soldiers with spinal injuries from war zone to hospital were a major source of bed sores, and poor treatment and poor care regimes allowed urinary infections to take hold. Those who survived, mostly previously active young men and women facing life as newly disabled people with numerous health problems, often became severely depressed and some attempted suicide.

Fig 7.5
Sir Ludwig Guttmann.
[Wikimedia Commons]

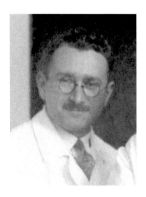

Guttmann was determined to tackle both the physical and mental rehabilitation of his young, paralysed charges. He had been forced to flee Germany with his family in 1939 because of the virulent Nazi persecution of the German Jewish population. Already recognised as a talented neurosurgeon keen to improve both medical and rehabilitative treatment of people who had suffered paralysing injuries, his move to Britain was supported by the British Society for the Protection of Science and Learning. Senior British medics, concerned about the low quality and poor outcomes of spinal injuries, asked Guttmann to report on his ideas for treatment and rehabilitation of peripheral nerve injury. They were so impressed with his theories that they asked him to put them into practice at the Stoke Mandeville Unit for the Spinal Injured in Aylesbury in southern England (Anderson 2011, 133–4; Wood 2011, 44–5).

The unit had opened in 1944 with just one ward and 28 beds. Both patients and staff were in a state of extreme low morale, with survival chances seen as minimal and prospects for any sort of happy or meaningful life after treatment virtually non-existent. Guttmann immediately introduced simple changes to the medical treatment regime which radically altered survival prospects. Standard mattresses were replaced with rubber ones, newly arrived patients were placed on 'pillow packs', patients were turned regularly in their beds, urinary systems were regularly disinfected, catheters were fitted, and supplies of penicillin were acquired to become a part of the treatment regime. All of this had a significant impact on physical patient health and survival prospects.

Yet Guttmann recognised that these depressed young people needed a rehabilitation system that paid attention to their minds as well as their bodies. Noting their competitive instincts and that most of them had led active lives before their disabling injuries, he began to introduce a regime of activities and sports, even when his patients were completely confined to bed in the initial stages of their treatment. They were given mirrors to enable them to ensure that they were sitting in an upright position to develop their upper body strength. As well as the dressing competitions, there would be simple activities such as throwing and catching a medicine ball between staff and patients, and equipment was introduced such as bed cycles, which could be positioned over a bed to enable a patient to exercise.

Competitive activity from the beds and the wards at Stoke Mandeville developed into darts, skittle and snooker competitions in local pubs. All of these could be played with relative ease from a wheelchair, and socialising with locals, who always welcomed them as heroes, was important for morale. Activities then progressed to wheelchair polo, shooting and archery. Games of wheelchair polo, in which teams used polo sticks to move the ball around, became so rough and competitive that they had to be replaced with the more sedate and non-contact sport of wheelchair netball. Guttmann's aim of bringing about reintegration through increased self-esteem and a sense of purpose was coming to fruition.

On 29 July 1948 – the opening day of the Olympic Games in London – an archery competition took place on the lawns of the hospital against a team from the Star and Garter residential home for war-disabled people in Richmond, Surrey. There were 16 competitors, including 2 women.

The success of the event prompted Guttmann to say afterwards: 'it was the first archery competition in the history of sport for the disabled. It was a demonstration to the public that competitive sport is not the prerogative of the able-bodied, but that the severely disabled, even those with paraplegia, can become sportsmen and women in their own right.' With these words Guttmann demonstrated his fierce commitment to moving from the model of pity he had first encountered when he walked into Stoke Mandeville to a new way of thinking in which disabled people could be confident of themselves and admired by others (Anderson 2011, 136–44; Wood 2011, 22–3).

In 1950 the games were named the Stoke Mandeville Festival of Sport and 10,000 people watched a wheelchair netball match at the Empress Hall in west London. People whose disabilities were caused by industrial accidents, many of them miners from the north of England, as well as military veterans, began to take part. In 1952 the games became international and by 1960 in Rome 400 disabled athletes from 22 countries were participating.

In 2001 Philip Craven became the president of the International Paralympics Committee. Paralysed aged 16 in a rock-climbing accident, he subsequently became one of the finest wheelchair basketball players in the world. Craven saw a need to change the way in which disability sport operated and was perceived. He was motivated not by the desire for medical rehabilitation but by a hunger to become a world-class elite player. For this new generation of disabled athletes it was time to turn away from what now appeared to be the anachronistic Guttmann medical model of sport as a form of treatment and confidence booster, to a new model of elite sporting activity by highly trained, skilled and professional athletes, who happened to be disabled. Led by him, the formidable Great Britain wheelchair basketball team became world champions in 1973.

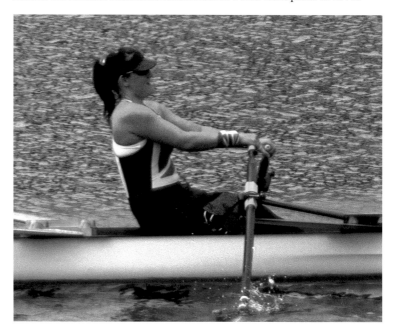

Fig 7.6
British Paralympian Sam
Scowen competes in the
mixed-double sculls at London
2012.
[www.flickr.com/photos/
thebarrowboy/7920514952/]

Under Craven, the transformation of the Paralympics, away from the idea of rehabilitation and towards the idea of world-class performance by elite athletes, gathered pace.

Today the Paralympics are one of the world's great international sporting events. At the 2012 London games 4,200 disabled athletes participated in 20 sports in a stunning range of fully accessible, 'universal design' venues (Fig 7.6). The games are no longer just about the rehabilitation of paralysed people; they are a global sports spectacle in their own right. Other famous sporting venues have opened up to disability sports, including Wimbledon, where wheelchair tennis is now played.

After the successful second games at Stoke Mandeville in 1949, Guttmann had made an optimistic speech, perhaps a little carried away by his enthusiasm, in which he said that the time would come when this, the Mandeville Games, would achieve world fame as the disabled person's equivalent of the Olympics (Wood 2011, 22). His dream, in a quiet corner of Buckinghamshire, has been realised in a way even he might not have imagined fully possible.

Mental health and the chemical solution

Sigmund Freud had died in 1939, in his home in Hampstead in London, the safe haven where this exile from the nightmare world of Nazism ended his days. The new way of thinking he had brought to the concept of the mind, his theories of the unconscious mental drives which exist in all humans, and which the talking cure of psychoanalysis could bring to the surface, lived on after him. However, psychoanalysis, after the Second World War, would face some challenges without him. It would come face to face with competing talking cures, such as the brief and more pragmatic interventions of Cognitive Behaviour Therapy (CBT), clinical psychology and therapeutic social work interventions. Private psychotherapists would offer sessions for individuals to talk through and attempt to resolve their mental conflicts, anxieties and depressive episodes. Psychoanalysis was no longer the overriding dominant model that it had staked a claim to be; it was now somewhat reduced, one among many, more impactful as a cultural phenomenon in the shared imagination of films, books and plays where psychoanalytic dramas loomed large, than in practice (Scull 2015, 380).

Psychoanalysis did, however, remain influential in the area of child psychology. In England the psychoanalysts John Bowlby, Donald Winnicot and Freud's daughter Anna pioneered a gentler manifestation of Freud's shocking sexual conflict theories to develop theories of attachment development (Fig 7.7). These theories provided a blueprint for supporting child–parent relations that could be happily adopted by the cautious and naturally conservative National Health Service (Scull 2015, 342).

Psychoanalysis had also given credence to the idea that mental ill health could affect anyone at any time, and was not confined to the certifiable mad of the institutions. Psychiatry, and the general public, now recognised that neuroses were widespread in the community at large, mostly not of an intensity requiring commitment to hospital but

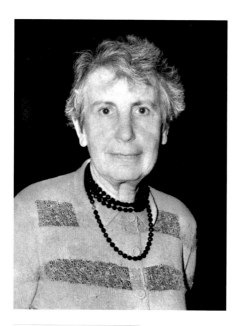

Fig 7.7

Anna Freud, a pioneer of child psychology, in 1957.

[Wikimedia Commons]

nevertheless a disturbance in the lives of many people at some point. The borderland between sanity and insanity could not be rigidly staked out by hospital walls, and the institution would never be a response to most people's needs. It was this understanding that drove a personalisation of management of mental health outside institutions and service networks in which many either purchased or were prescribed a talking intervention to seek mental equilibrium (Porter 2002, 208–9).

Nevertheless, outside the low-level interactions of the therapist's room, many people with mental illness were still locked up, institutionalised and isolated. In the 1950s in England and Wales more than 150,000 people were still confined in mental hospitals at any given time throughout the decade. The hospitals had been, since 1948, under the control of the new National Health Service, but this did not bring the people in them the improvements and new-found optimism that the NHS was bringing to the rest of the population (Scull 2015, 362).

Mental hospitals, their staff, and their patients drifted aimlessly. It needed a social policy revolution to change them, and in England this came in the surprising form of Enoch Powell, Minister of Health in the Conservative Macmillan government. In a speech addressed to the National Association of Mental Health conference in 1961, which has become known as the 'water towers' speech, he denounced the remnants of the Victorian asylum system which the hospitals represented:

> There they stand, isolated, majestic, imperious, brooded over by the gigantic water tower and chimney combined, rising unmistakable and daunting out of the countryside – the asylums which our forefathers built with such immense solidity – to express the notions of their day.
>
> (Nuffield Trust)

Powell promised a shift to community-based services which would mirror those for physical health in the wider health care system, where hospital was only a place for the most acutely ill. A system of community psychiatrists and nurses, day wards and community-based services would replace the institutions. Shortly after Powell's speech the long-stay hospitals were informed that they would receive no further upgrading or refurbishment, as within 10 to 15 years they would not be required. It would, in fact, be the 1990s before they were fully closed, but their death knell had sounded that day in 1961 (Fig 7.8).

The right-wing libertarian instincts of Powell were part of an unlikely alliance between the right, who saw mental hospitals as both an expensive waste of resources and an exemplar of excessive state control over the lives of individuals, and leftist critiques of psychiatry and its coercive practices. In the same year as Powell's speech, in the United States the sociologist Erving Goffman published his *Asylums: Essays on the Social Situation of Mental Patients and Other Inmates*, which denounced mental hospitals as 'total institutions' that degraded and caused massive

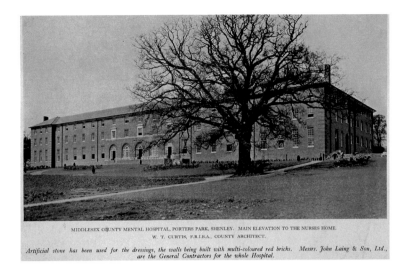

MIDDLESEX COUNTY MENTAL HOSPITAL, PORTERS PARK, SHENLEY. MAIN ELEVATION TO THE NURSES HOME.
W. T. CURTIS, F.R.I.B.A., COUNTY ARCHITECT.

*Artificial stone has been used for the dressings, the walls being built with multi-coloured red bricks. Messrs. John Laing & Son, Ltd.,
are the General Contractors for the whole Hospital.*

Fig 7.8
Enoch Powell described the
mental hospital as 'isolated,
majestic, imperious' – Shenley
Hospital in Hertfordshire.
[Wellcome Collection]

damage to the people confined within them. The apparently pathological
behaviours of patients were in large part rational responses to the
degradations that were inflicted on them.

In the United Kingdom the Marxist Scottish psychiatrist R D
Laing began what became known as the 'anti-psychiatry movement'
(Fig 7.9). Laing saw mental illness as real, but argued that madness
was the product of society, particularly family relationships. Laing, like
Goffman, saw the mental hospital as a deeply destructive environment.
The proper place for patients locked up in such hospitals was the
community, where they should be coaxed to complete their therapeutic
journey, rather than institutionalised and drugged into submission
(Scull 2015, 573–4).

Fig 7.9
The psychiatrist R D Laing
questioned the basic precepts
of psychiatry.
[Robert E Hareldsen]

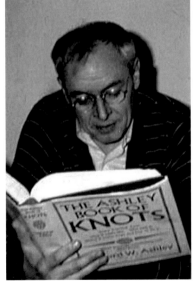

Laing's reference to drugs was significant, because the
post-war period was also the time of the so-called chemical
revolution. Interest in psychopharmacology, and the ability
of drugs to alter, control or cure the moods and behaviours of
people with mental illness, rose sharply. The first psychotropic,
or mood influencing, drug was introduced in 1949. In the 1950s
drug companies developed anti-psychotic and anti-depressant
drugs such as chlorpromazine (or Largactil) and imipramine.
The powerful effects of these drugs in reducing psychotic
or depressive episodes were unmistakable, and the British
psychiatrist William Sargent, who pursued psychosurgery and
electroconvulsive and insulin shock therapies with evangelical
zeal, crowed that they would deliver mental patients not only
from the asylum but also what he saw as the foolishness of
psychoanalysis, which he referred to as 'cackle'. But there were
other effects too. Largactil became known as the 'chemical
cosh', reducing its recipients to pitiful shadows of their former
selves. Other mood-altering drugs had similar effects. The
journalist Martin Townsend, in his memoir of life with his
mentally ill father, recalled a hospital doctor's discussion with
his mother about his father's lithium dosage:

'It's not a good drug', one of the doctors told my mum one afternoon. 'It's a drug that causes terrible side-effects – the knee jerks, the twitching, the lips all that … we just have to find a way, long-term, of bringing the dose right down. Physically it is not doing him any good at all.'

(Townsend 2007, 262)

The price of chemical intervention as an alternative to institutionalisation, for many, was becoming all too clear. Townsend described a visit to his father when the effects of his medication were painfully apparent:

His mouth was trembling in a very strange way and there was dribble on his lips … His eyes seemed to be glazed and tearful … As he came close I could see that his arms and hands were also trembling. His hands seemed elongated … His legs were shaking too.

'Are you OK Dad?' I said.

'Yeah, no. I'm alright,' he said. He half-raised his arm. His voice seemed slurry … as if he had a heavy cold. 'It's just the drugs.' He slurred the 'just the' so it came out as 'sus-de'.

(Townsend 2007, 125–6)

Psychotropic drugs certainly offered an alternative to devastating brain surgery, asylums and the psychoanalysis that was out of the financial reach of most, but often came at a cost.

New drugs enjoyed phenomenal success, and their use extended far beyond the certifiable patient. The tranquiliser Valium (diazepam) became the most widely prescribed medication in the 1960s, and from 1987 Prozac, which was claimed to lift mood by raising serotonin levels, was being prescribed to millions worldwide. Once more hopes were raised, as they had been for centuries, that there was a cure, a solution, for those whose minds were not at rest (Porter 2002, 205–7).

Back to the community – disability equality, rights and inclusion

In 1951 800 people took part in a 'silent reproach' march to Downing Street. They were members of the British Limbless Ex-Servicemen's Association, protesting that their pensions had dropped below the cost of living. They were to protest again in 1956. In 1946 a letter in the *National Cripples' Journal* had lambasted the government's promise of 'security from cradle to grave', claiming that while disabled ex-servicemen, the elderly, the blind and those injured in industrial accidents were all supported with pensions under the new cradle-to-grave welfare state, it did nothing for 'the civilian cripple, who is incapable of earning a living'. There was a new militancy in the air. If there was going to be a bold new society fit for all, disabled people must be a part of that 'all' (Anderson 2011, 189).

A host of new campaigning organisations sprang up. In 1946 The National Association for Mental Health and the National Association of Parents of Backward Children formed, later becoming MIND and Mencap respectively. The Leonard Cheshire Foundation, British Epilepsy Association, the Spastics Society (now Scope), and hundreds of others soon followed. Parents were often the instigators of these new civil organisations, tired of seeing their sons and daughters excluded from education as children and then employment or support when they became adults.

The National Association of Parents of Backward Children was formed by young mother Judy Fryd, and was to a large extent a challenge to medical authority, a counterpoint to doctors who told parents of disabled newborns to have them taken into the care of long-stay hospitals, forget they had been born, and try for another child. Eugenics may have been exposed as a shameful and murderous cult by events in Nazi Germany, but eugenic thinking did not disappear from the medical profession. It was re-presented in disguised, softer forms, as concern for the family who had borne a child with a disability, and 'genetic counselling'. The battle therefore was to gain recognition for children and adults with disabilities as people, not as some form of not-quite-human burden. As one parent activist put it:

> [We] were trying to get support and recognition as much as anything, to try and get people to treat our people as though there was at least a certain amount of normality. They were all human beings … And also to try and get the children, although they weren't children all of them, recognised as people.
>
> (Rolph *et al* 2005, 78)

There was a growing unwillingness to defer passively to medical opinion. Parents fought for a new community-based system of support to challenge the institutional hospital behemoth. They lobbied for the right of every child to receive an education and campaigned for nurseries, occupational centres, youth clubs, respite and residential homes, sometimes establishing them through their own efforts (Jarrett 2020, 286).

In Parliament, disabled MPs led the struggle for the rights of people with physical disabilities. Two wounded First World War veterans, the double amputee Jack Brunel-Cohen (Liverpool Fairfield) and the blinded Ian Fraser (Morecambe and Lonsdale, Lancaster), fought for disabled servicemen's rights. The deaf MP Jack Ashley (Stoke-on-Trent South) campaigned for the rights of disabled people generally.

Following on from the parent-led organisations of the late 1940s and early 1950s, campaigning organisations formed and led by disabled people themselves came to the fore in the 1970s, drawing inspiration from the wider civil rights movement. After DIG's 1960s campaign for improved disablement benefits (and in part frustrated by DIG's limited aims), the Union of the Physically Impaired Against Segregation (UPIAS) was established in 1972 by disabled activists Paul Hunt and Vik Finkelstein, whose campaigning objective was for disabled people to be able to take control of their own lives rather than have them controlled by others. In their founding statement they announced:

We reject also the whole idea of 'experts' and professionals holding forth on how we should accept our disabilities, or giving learned lectures about the 'psychology' of disablement. We already know what it feels like to be poor, isolated, segregated, done good to, stared at, and talked down to – far better than any non-disabled expert. We as a Union are not interested in descriptions of how awful it is to be disabled. What we are interested in, are ways of changing our conditions of life, and thus overcoming the disabilities which are imposed on to our physical impairments by the way this society is organised to exclude us. In our view, it is only the actual impairment which we must accept; the additional and totally unnecessary problems caused by the way we are treated are essentially to be overcome and not accepted. We look forward to the day when the army of 'experts' on our social and psychological problems can find more productive work.

(Oliver and Barnes 1998, 109)

While UPIAS was Marxist-inspired, the Disability Alliance, formed in 1974 and chaired by the academic Peter Townsend, was a cross-impairment reformist movement seeking to bring together a coalition of disability groups, disabled individuals and non-disabled academics and experts. Like UPIAS, the Disability Alliance was underpinned by the social model, but like DIG focused on poverty as the fundamental issue causing the segregation and exclusion of disabled people. UPIAS saw itself as campaigning on a wider range of issues and having a wider theoretical critique of the disablement imposed by society on physically impaired people (Shakespeare 2014, 14–16).

The Mental Patients Union (MPU) was founded in 1973 at Paddington Day Hospital in London by a group of six patients. Among their demands were the abolition of compulsory treatment, with patients having the right to refuse any specific treatment. They also demanded the abolition of the right of any authorities to treat patients in the face of opposition of relatives or closest friends unless the patient of their own volition desired the treatment. Finally, they advocated the abolition of irreversible psychiatric treatments such as electroconvulsive therapy (ECT), brain surgery, and certain drugs.

The People First movement, a self-advocacy group formed of people with learning disabilities, began at the Fairview Training Centre in Oregon USA in the 1970s and started in the UK in 1984. It campaigns to this day for equal citizenship for people with learning disabilities.

New thinking drove these activist alliances. In 1968 the American academic Wolf Wolfensberger had first set out his creed denouncing asylums and long-stay hospitals as abusive institutions which dehumanised people through their design and their routines. Wolfensberger argued that institutions were built around models of seeing 'retarded' persons that stripped them of their personhood (Wolfensberger 1975, 13–15).

Disabled campaigners, such as the sociologist Michael Oliver and disability studies pioneer Vic Finkelstein at the Open University, advocated the social model of disability as one in which disabled people could control their own lives, challenging the attitudes of non-disabled society. They framed the struggle of disabled people to be included as a fight against society, not against their own bodies. Disability, and the exclusion that accompanies it, is 'constructed' because society chooses to see it that way, rather than being an inevitable consequence of physical bodily impairment. They argued for a world 'where impairment is valued and celebrated and all disabling barriers are eradicated. Such a world would be inclusionary for all' (Oliver and Barnes 1998, 102).

Despite all this campaigning activity, post-war, long-stay hospitals for people with learning disabilities or mental illness seemed neglected and forgotten. From the 1960s, abuse scandals erupted onto newspaper front pages, triggering enquiries at Farleigh Hospital in Flax Bourton, Somerset, and Coldharbour in Sherborne, Dorset. There were discoveries (usually by journalists) of major abuse across the NHS in Britain: at Ely hospital in Cardiff (1967), South Ockenden in Essex (1974), and Normansfield in south London (1976). In 1981 an infamous television documentary, *Silent Minority*, exposed further scandals at St Lawrence's in Caterham, Surrey, and Borocourt in Reading, Berkshire. Public disquiet became overwhelming. The 1981 Care in the Community Green Paper signalled the end of the asylum. Over the following two decades tens of thousands of people moved from hospitals back to the community. The old hospitals breathed their last as institutions, marking finally an end to the asylum era that had begun in the early 19th century. A new era of residential and group homes, day-care facilities and independent living within mainstream communities began. It was the end of the long-stay Victorian institution but not necessarily an end to the perceptions and practices of institutionalisation (Fig 7.10).

Many benefited and flourished as the return to the community took place (Fig 7.11). However, there was always a sense that, for some, real freedom and real belonging were elusive. The place of people

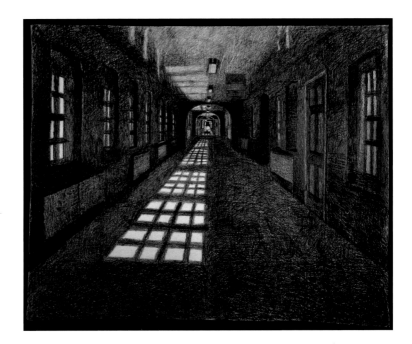

Fig 7.10
End of the asylum? A drawing of High Royds Hospital in Yorkshire, made in 2003 shortly before its closure. [Wellcome Collection. Attribution 4.0 International (CC by 4.0)]

Fig 7.11
Many have benefited and
flourished as a result of the
return to the community.
These young people with
Down syndrome can now live
their lives.
[Wellcome Collection.
Attribution 4.0 International
(CC by 4.0)]

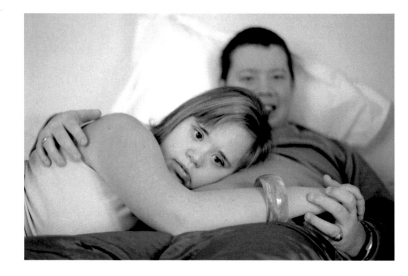

within communities could feel at times conditional, dependent on their
conformity to the norms and expectations of the rest of society. Small-
group living and community-based services could be in subtle ways just
as isolating as institutional life. People could be *in* their communities but
not be *of* them, an invisible bureaucratic wall of professional control and
service-led practice replacing the more visible asylum wall to drive a sense
of isolation.

Ideas continue to change. In the 21st century, notions of
empowerment and self-direction, where disabled people control their
own service budgets to buy support, rather than 'receiving' care, have
come to the fore. The idea of specialist homes and buildings is challenged
in favour of universal design and buildings. We find ourselves at the end
of the asylum period, an era which in the end only represents 150 years
of disability history and which never involved all disabled people. But for
how long will the shadow of Bedlam continue to be cast? Pressures on
public finances have led to a slow return of larger group housing projects,
away from more independent living. 'Assessment and Treatment Centres',
looking suspiciously like long-stay hospitals despite ostensibly only
admitting people for short periods of time (just as asylum advocates once
promised would happen), incarcerate at the time of writing more than

Fig 7.12
The struggle goes on –
disability protests in Norfolk
2015.
[Roger Blackwell]

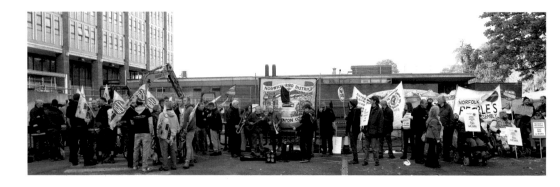

2,000 people with learning disabilities or autism, deemed 'challenging'. Some have remained in these institutions for more than 20 years. Benefits and other forms of support, including employment support, which have enabled disabled people to lead the lives they wish, have been reduced. Despite many advances and much progress, there is rising anxiety that the institution may not have been killed off, and may be stirring again – the future remains uncertain (Fig 7.12).

Conclusion

The extermination project against disabled people by the Nazi party in Germany from 1939 to 1941 during the Second World War marks probably the darkest moment in the history of disabled people, a history which has had many dark moments, particularly in the last two centuries. It was in some ways a logical culmination of eugenic ideas, in which the unfit are bred out of society and only the healthy remain. Much of the 20th century, even setting aside the Nazi horrors, can be marked down as a period of mass libel and indictment against disabled people, who were often seen as culpable for the 'difference' of their bodies and minds, a stain and a threat to order, progress and civilisation. Eugenic science, despite being predicated on falsity, distortion and moral incoherence, became part of the normative assumptions of many Western societies. The hostility and malice directed at disabled people from powerful medical, scientific, intellectual and political groups was mixed in with racial and social anxieties about the end of civilisation, the imperative for progress, and the quest for perfection. In their most extreme form, in parts of Europe, these anxieties were played out in the totalitarian movements of fascism and communism. Fascism had no place for disabled people in its racialised Aryan fantasy; communism saw no need for them in the socially perfectionist utopia it was building.

The latter half of the century saw a turn for the better, as asylums closed, legislation outlawed discrimination and universal rights declarations were issued. Such moves are improvements indeed, but are also reminders of the deep discrimination and anti-disability sentiments that made them necessary in the first place. Declaring rights does not ensure rights, outlawing discrimination does not abolish discrimination, and acknowledging former wrongs does not mean that wrongs disappear. Societies still carry within them the shadow of what has gone before. The story of the 20th century is also a reminder to us modern people that we should never look back on the past with condescending eyes and view history as a linear narrative of progress towards the achievements of now. No century offered such a bleak and cruel existence to so many disabled people as the supposedly sophisticated 20th century. More enlightened thinking on disability was offered in the medieval and early modern periods than most modern intellectuals have ever managed to achieve.

Yet through the libels and the indictments, disabled people soldiered on (literally in some cases) and fought the battle for acceptance, inclusion, change and opportunity that they have always fought. That fight will never stop.

Discussion: Rights and self-representation

The 20th century saw the growth of the disability rights movement which challenged conventional thinking on disability. But this was not the only time when disabled people spoke up for themselves. How have people seen themselves, and described themselves, over the centuries?

There is a view of a person with a disability, perhaps owing much to 19th-century writers, which sees them as a hapless victim, with little to say for themselves, and hopelessly dependent on the goodwill and beneficence of others. The chief proponent of this sort of sentimental and cloying portrayal (as discussed in Chapter 5, p 98) was the novelist Charles Dickens, whose 'Tiny Tim' Cratchit character in *A Christmas Carol* (1843) epitomises the voiceless passivity of this strain of the Victorian depiction of disability. Tiny Tim's only memorable words are 'God bless us every one', as the boy, probably affected by rickets, waits helplessly for a transformation in Scrooge's social attitudes to save his life. Such sentimentality in the depiction of the passive disabled person was by no means confined to Dickens and can be found across the art and literature of the Victorian period.

Nor did such characterisations of disability disappear once the Victorian era ended. Until the 1980s, the campaigning charity Mencap used the image of 'little Stephen', a helpless and sad-looking learning-disabled child, and the Spastics Society (now Scope) used as a collecting box a similarly sad-looking girl with a calliper. Campaigners at the time from these two groups might have argued that pity and sympathy were a better deal than being completely frozen out of people's minds altogether and left to rot in an asylum. However, such imagery perpetuated the idea of passivity and suffering, and of a life over which the disabled person had no control.

The idea of disabled people as passive, as objects or functions of other people's actions and beliefs, is a strong one. It is prominent in the medical model of disability, where they can be seen as little more than a body which needs fixing or improving. It is also evident in some Christian and modern secular narratives of disability in which a person with a disability is seen as one who suffers, bravely or otherwise. It is easy to see what Wolf Wolfensberger was talking about when he referred to the power of conceptions of disability that portray the disabled person as sick, an object of pity, a holy innocent or a burden of charity (Wolfensberger 1975). Tim Cratchit, young and tiny as he is, is made to carry the weight of all these formulations of disability by Charles Dickens. The disability theorists Sharon L Snyder and David T Mitchell called such roles in fiction, film and art a 'narrative prosthesis', where the disabled person is used as a metaphorical crutch to carry a storyline to a particular conclusion. These characters have no depth or complexity of character themselves, but are used in a highly symbolic way to throw light on other, non-disabled characters (Mitchell and Snyder 2000). This type of disability symbolism is evident in *Rain Man*, the 1988 movie in which the selfish, self-absorbed Charlie Babbit (Tom Cruise) is brought to a state of enlightenment and self-improvement simply by being in the presence of his 'autistic savant' brother Raymond (Dustin Hoffman). The role of Raymond Babbit is a symbolic one, to affect and bring about change in what can appear to be the more important non-disabled characters around him, rather than be a rounded character in his own right.

Such portrayals, and the political development of the disability rights movements since the latter part of the 20th century, might suggest to us that the phenomenon of disabled people standing up for their rights and being political actors in their own lives is a relatively recent one. However, this is an inaccurate framing of history. Far from being passive victims, there are numerous examples in history of disabled people standing up for and asserting themselves in all walks of life. As we saw in Chapter 2, in the late 13th century the residents of the leper house in the Norfolk village of West Somerton mutinied against the oppressive and thieving clerical gang running the institution, looting and demolishing the buildings and killing the prior's guard dog. They won the resulting court case with the jury taking their side and the prior was instructed to enact urgent reforms. In the face of oppression, they became agents of their own destinies and fought a winning battle.

While much art which features representations of disability resorts to characterisations of pity or menace where characters with disabilities are given a highly symbolic role, there are other representations which paint a very different picture. In William Hogarth's satirical series 'Humours of an Election' from 1755, the riotous painting *Chairing the Member* depicts an enormous brawl breaking out between rival political factions while the victorious newly elected MP is about to fall from the chair on which he is being paraded around in celebration. In the foreground and at the heart of the brawl stands a one-legged sailor engaged in a ferocious cudgel fight with a political opponent. The sailor's wooden prosthetic leg is placed firmly on the ground balancing him while he trades blows. His posture is heroic and muscular, his disability a side issue, his position an equal one with his non-disabled opponent (Figs 7.13 and 7.14). Other crowd scenes by Hogarth depict disability in 18th-century England in a similarly active, if not always flattering, formulation. In the background of his famous *Gin Lane* print of 1751, which depicted the depravities brought about by gin consumption in London, crutches and sticks fly though the air in the background as drunken crowds engage in a mass fight. There are no Tiny Tims to be seen. This other narrative, of independence and self-assertion, has always been in evidence. As the stories in Chapter 6 about disabled children resisting brutality and abusive treatment in 20th-century special schools reveal, even in the atmosphere of loathing and hostility towards those with disabilities by some people at certain times, disabled people have always stood firm in some way and taken action to resist both the metaphorical and actual straitjackets into which society was trying to bind them.

As the concept of 'disability' developed over the 20th century into a term to describe all types of impairment, sensory, bodily and mental, so rights movements began to coalesce around the concept, as exclusion and discrimination widened into political rather than personal issues. The limbless ex-serviceman's silent march of reproach in London in 1951 symbolised this emerging politicised dynamic as disabled people saw

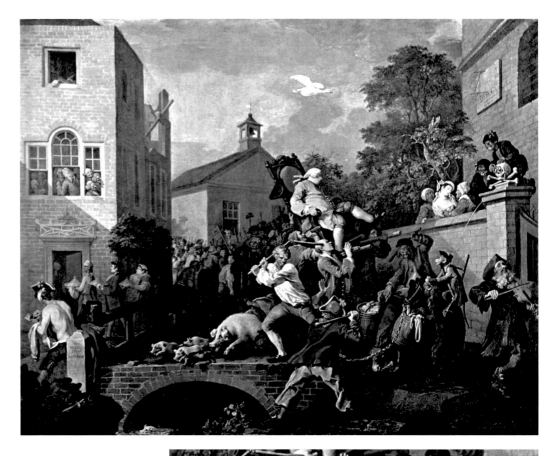

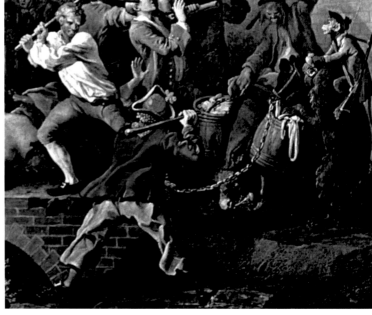

Fig 7.13
In Hogarth's scene we see a
sailor with one leg fighting
during a political riot.
[DIRECTMEDIA]

Fig 7.14
Heroic posture – Hogarth's
fighting sailor.
[DIRECTMEDIA]

themselves as excluded from many of the benefits brought by the new welfare state to their non-disabled counterparts in British society. The disability rights movement from the 1970s, inspired by the wider global civil rights movement, marked the full flowering of this political turn. However, these political movements built on a legacy of disabled people over many centuries refusing to accept the passive or pitiful roles which many tried to assign to them, and fighting for their status, however much the odds were stacked against them.

Bibliography

Anderson, J 2011 *War, Disability and Rehabilitation in Britain: 'Soul of a Nation'*. Manchester: Manchester University Press

Andrews, J 1996 'Identifying and Providing for the Mentally Disabled in Early Modern London' *in* A Digby and D Wright (eds), *From Idiocy to Mental Deficiency: Historical Perspectives on People with Learning Disabilities*. London: Routledge, 65–92

Andrews, J, and Scull, A 2003 *Customers and Patrons of the Mad-Trade: The Management of Lunacy in 18th-Century London*. Berkeley: University of California Press

Andrews J, Briggs, A, Porter R, Tucker P, and Waddington, K 1997 *The History of Bethlem*. Abingdon: Routledge

Anon nd *The Merry Miscellany*. Bristol

Atkinson, D, Jackson, M, and Walmsley, J 1997 *Forgotten Lives: Exploring the History of Learning Disability*. Kidderminster: BILD

Bailey, B 1988 *Almshouses*. London: Robert Hale

Beier, A L 1985 *Masterless Men: The Vagrancy Problem in England 1560–1640*. London: Methuen

Borsay, A 2005 *Disability and Social Policy in Britain since 1750: A History of Exclusion*. Basingstoke: Palgrave Macmillan

Chambers, P 2009 *Bedlam: London's Hospital for the Mad*. Hersham: Ian Allen

Chatelet, A M, Lerch, D, and Luc, J-N 2003 *Ecole de Plein Air (Open Air Schools)*. Paris: Editions Recherches

Clay, R 1909 *The Mediaeval Hospitals of England*. London: Methuen

Cruikshank, C G 1968 *Elizabeth's Army*. Oxford: Oxford University Press

Curtis, B, and Thompson, S 2014 '"A Plentiful Crop of Cripples Made by all This Progress": Disability, Artificial Limbs and Working Class Mutualism in the South Wales Coalfield, 1890–1948'. *Social History of Medicine* 27:4, 708–27

Englander, D 1998 *Poverty and Poor Law Reform in 19th Century Britain, 1834–1914: From Chadwick to Booth*. London: Longman

Forbes, T R 1971 *Chronicle from Aldgate: Life and Death in Shakespeare's London*. New Haven: Yale University Press

Frith, U 1989 *Autism: Explaining the Enigma*. Oxford: Blackwell

Gilbert, M 1995 *The First World War*. London: Harper Collins

Gladstone, D 1996 'The Changing Dynamic of Institutional Care: The Western Counties Idiot Asylum 1864–1914' *in* A Digby and D Wright (eds) *From Idiocy to Mental Deficiency: Historical Perspectives on People with Learning Disabilities*. London: Routledge, 134–60

Goffman, E 1961 *Asylums: Essays on the Social Situation of Mental Patients and Other Inmates*. London: Penguin

Goldman, L 2006 'Fawcett, Henry (1833–1884), Economist and Politician'. *Oxford Dictionary of National Biography*. Retrieved 18 March 2021 from https://doi.org/10.1093/ref:odnb/9218

Goldsmith, S 1963 *Designing for the Disabled: A Manual of Technical Information*. London: Royal Institute of British Architects

Goldsmith, S 1997 *Designing for the Disabled: The New Paradigm*. London: Architectural Press

Gough, R 1988 *The History of Myddle*. London: Penguin

Hallett, A 2004 *Almshouses*. Princes Risborough: Shire

Harman, T 1972 'A Caveat for Common Cursitors', *in* G Salgado (ed), *Coney Catchers and Bawdey Baskets: An Anthology of Elizabethan Low Life*. London: Penguin, 79–154

Hitchcock, T 2004 *Down and Out in 18th-Century London*. London: Hambledon and London

Humphries, S, and Gordon, P 1992 *Out of Sight: The Experience of Disability 1900–1950*. Plymouth: Northcote House

Jackson, P, and Lee, R 2001 *Deaf Lives: Deaf People in History*. Feltham: British Deaf History Society

Jackson, R (ed) 2006 *Holistic Special Education: Camphill Principles and Practices*. Edinburgh: Floris

Jackson, R 2008 'The Camphill Movement: The Moravian Dimension'. *Journal of Moravian History* 5, 2008, 89–100

Jackson, R (ed) 2011 *Discovering Camphill: New Perspectives, Research and Developments*. Edinburgh: Floris

Jackson, R 2011 'The Origin of Camphill and the Social Pedagogic Impulse'. *Educational Review* 63:1, 95–104

Jarrett, S 2020 *Those They Called Idiots: The Idea of the Disabled Mind from 1700 to the Present Day*. London: Reaktion

Jordan, W K 1960 *The Charities of London 1480–1660: The Aspirations and the Achievements of the Urban Society*. London: Allen and Unwin

Kelly, S 2021 'We Should be Proud of Who We Are: Interview with Jane Campbell'. *Community Living* 34:3, 18–19

König, K 1960 *The Camphill Movement*. Whitby: Camphill Press

Longmate, N 2003 *The Workhouse: A Social History*. London: Pimlico

McIntyre, L 2015 'Goldsmith, (Philip) Selwyn (1932–2011), Architect'. *Oxford Dictionary of National Biography*. Retrieved 1 April 2021 from https://www-oxforddnb-com.ezproxy.lib.bbk.ac.uk/view/10.1093/ref:odnb/9780198614128.001.0001/odnb-9780198614128-e-103616

MacDonald, M 1981 *Mystical Bedlam: Madness, Anxiety and Healing in 17th-Century England*. Cambridge: Cambridge University Press

Mantin, M 2009 *'A Great Army of Suffering Ones': The Guild of the Brave Poor Things and Disability in the Late 19th and Early 20th Centuries*. Bristol: University of Bristol, Dept of Historical Studies

May, T 2011 *The Victorian Workhouse*. Oxford: Shire

Metzler, I 2006 *Disability in Medieval Europe: Thinking about Physical Impairment during the High Middle Ages*. Abingdon: Routledge

Metzler, I 2013 *A Social History of Disability in the Middle Ages: Cultural Considerations of Physical Impairment*. Abingdon: Routledge

Metzler, I 2016 *Fools and Idiots? Intellectual Disability in the Middle Ages*. Manchester: Manchester University Press

Mitchell, D T, and Snyder, S L 2000 *Narrative Prosthesis: Disability and the Dependencies of Discourse*. Ann Arbor: University of Michigan Press

Mortimer, F L 1848 *The Cripple*. London: John Hatfield and Son

Mounsey, C 2019 *Sight Correction: Vision and Blindness in 18th-Century Britain*. Charlottesville: University of Virginia Press

Nuffield Trust, National Health Service History, Enoch Powell, THE RT. HON. J. ENOCH POWELL, Minister of Health, Address to the National Association of Mental Health Annual Conference, 9 March 1961. www.nuffieldtrust.org.uk/files/2019-11/nhs-history-book/58-67/powell-s-water-tower-speech.html (accessed 8 April 2021)

OBP [Old Bailey Papers] 1710, Trial of Mary Bradshaw alias Seymour (t17011206-22)

Oliver, M 1990 *The Politics of Disablement*. Basingstoke: Macmillan

Oliver, M, and Barnes, C 1998 *Disabled People and Social Policy: From Exclusion to Inclusion*. London: Longman

Orme, N, and Webster, M 1995 *The English Hospital 1070–1570*. Newhaven: Yale University Press

Overy, R 2010 *The Morbid Age: Britain and the Crisis of Civilization, 1919–1939*. London: Penguin

Parry-Jones, W 1972 *The Trade in Lunacy: A Study of Private Madhouses in England in the 18th and 19th Centuries*. London: Routledge

Pelling, M 1998 *The Common Lot: Sickness, Medical Occupations and the Urban Poor in Early Modern England*. Harlow: Longman

Phillips, G 2006 (May 25) 'Armitage, Thomas Rhodes (1824–1890), Campaigner for Blind People'. *Oxford Dictionary of National Biography*. Retrieved 18 March 2021 from www-oxforddnb-com.ezproxy.lib.bbk.ac.uk/view/10.1093/ref:odnb/9780198614128.001.0001/odnb-9780198614128-e-62508

Porter, R 1992 'Madness and Its Institutions' *in* A Wear (ed) *Medicine in Society: Historical Essays*. Cambridge: Cambridge University Press, 277–302

Porter, R 2002 *Madness: A Brief History*. Oxford: Oxford University Press

Pound, J F 1971 *The Norwich Census of the Poor 1570*. Norwich: Norfolk Record Society

Quennel, P (ed) 1987 *Mayhew's London Underworld*. London: Century

Rawcliffe, C 2006 *Leprosy in Medieval England*. Woodbridge: Boydell

Reeves, C 2011 'Everyday Life for Jewish Patients in Colney Hatch', *Shemot* 19:3, 1–2, 33

Roberts, A (nd) Mental Health History Timeline. http://studymore.org.uk/mhhtim.htm

Rodger, N A M 1986 *The Wooden World: An Anatomy of the Georgian Navy*. London: Fontana

Rolph, S, Atkinson, D, Nind, M, and Welshman, J 2005 *Witnesses to Change: Families, Learning Difficulties and History*. Kidderminster: BILD

Rushton, P 1996 'Idiocy, the Family and the Community in Early Modern North-East England' *in* A Digby and D Wright (eds), *From Idiocy to Mental Deficiency: Historical Perspectives on People with Learning Disabilities*. London: Routledge, 44–64

Rutherford, S 2010 *The Victorian Asylum*. Oxford: Shire

Safford, P L, and Safford, E J 1996 *A History of Childhood and Disability*. New York: Teachers College Press

Scull, A 1980 'A Convenient Place to Get Rid of Inconvenient People: The Victorian Lunatic Asylum' *in* A D King (ed) *Buildings and Society: Essays on the Social Development of the Built Environment*. London: Routledge and Keegan Paul, 37–60

Scull, A 1993 *The Most Solitary of Afflictions: Madness and Society in Britain, 1700–1900*. New Haven: Yale University Press

Scull, A 2015 *Madness in Civilization: A Cultural History of Insanity from the Bible to Freud, From the Madhouse to Modern Medicine*. London: Thames and Hudson

Scull, A, MacKenzie, C, and Hervey, N 1996 *Masters of Bedlam: The Transformation of the Mad-Doctoring Trade*. Princeton, NJ: Princeton University Press

Segal, S (ed) 1990 *The Place of Special Villages and Residential Communities*. Bicester: A B Academic

Shakespeare, T 2006 *Disability Rights and Wrongs*. Abingdon: Routledge

Shakespeare, T 2014 *Disability Rights and Wrongs Revisited*. Abingdon: Routledge

Sheffer, E 2018 *Asperger's Children: The Origins of Autism in Nazi Vienna*. New York: Norton

Slack, P 1995 *The English Poor Law, 1531–1782*. Cambridge: Cambridge University Press

Southworth, J 2003 *Fools and Jesters at the English Court*. Stroud: Sutton

Stevenson, C 2000 *Medicine and Magnificence: British Hospital and Asylum Architecture 1660–1815*. New Haven, CT: Yale University Press

Strype, J 1816 *Ecclesiastical Memorials: Relating Chiefly to Religion, and Its Reformation Under the Reigns of King Henry VIII*. London: Bagster

The National Archives (TNA) MH12/9530/338 (Southwell 341)

The National Archives (TNA) MH51/44B Liverpool Lunatic Asylum Laws and Rules 1834 and Buckinghamshire County Pauper Lunatic Asylum General Rules 1854

The National Archives (TNA) MH58/97 Board of Control Committee on Mental Deficiency Colonies. Hedley Committee Report January 1930

The National Archives (TNA) NATS 1/727 Central Association for the Care of the Mentally Defective: Request for information regarding rejection of soldiers for mental deficiency 1917–18. Letter from Sir Leslie Scott 23 November 1917

The National Archives (TNA) 1926 RG48/159 Proposed marriage of adult mental defective

Townsend, M 2007 *The Father I Had*. Corgi: London

Trenery, C 2019 *Madness, Medicine and Miracle in Twelfth-Century England*. Abingdon: Routledge

Turner, D 2012 *Disability in 18th-Century England: Imagining Physical Impairment*. London: Routledge

Turner, D, and Blackie, D 2018 *Disability in the Industrial Revolution: Physical Impairment in British Coalmining, 1780–1880*. Manchester: Manchester University Press

Turner, W 2018 'Conceptualization of Intellectual Disability in Medieval English Law', *in* P McDonagh, C F Goodey, and T Stainton (eds) *Intellectual Disability: A Conceptual History, 1200–1900*. Manchester: Manchester University Press, 26–44

Wolfensberger, W 1975 *The Origin and Nature of our Institutionalized Models*. New York: Human Policy Press

Wood, C 2011 *The True Story of Great Britain's Paralympic Heroes*. London: Carlton

Wright, D 2001 *Mental Disability in Victorian England: The Earlswood Asylum 1847–1901*. Oxford: Clarendon Press

Wynter, A 1870 'Non-restraint in Treatment of the Insane'. *Edinburgh Review*, 131

Glossary

access/accessibility The features of a building or area such as ramps, sliding doors, toilets etc which ensure that it can be used by disabled people.

airing court A walled garden area leading off from 19th-century asylum wards where patients were allowed to exercise and 'take the air' without risk of 'escape'. Often contained shelters and ornamental features.

alienist The early 19th-century word for the medical professional who would later become known as a psychiatrist.

alms Charitable donations of food or money to the poor or those considered unable to look after themselves.

alms givers Those who give alms to the needy.

almshouses Homes built, from the medieval period onwards, to shelter elderly, disabled or other people considered unable to look after themselves. Sometimes known as 'Maisons Dieu'.

ambulant disabled People who have a disability but are able to walk and do not use a wheelchair.

Asperger syndrome The name given for a form of autism which particularly affects communication and interaction with others, and the anxiety levels caused by communication. Named after controversial Austrian physician Hans Asperger, who worked in Vienna during the Nazi period. The diagnosis was removed in 2013 from the DSM-5 (Diagnostic and Statistical Manual of Mental Disorders) and incorporated into the range known as autistic spectrum disorder.

asylum Form of institution particularly for mentally ill or learning-disabled people which creates a fully segregated environment set apart from mainstream society. Began as charitable institutions in England in late 18th century, built and provided by the state from 1815.

attendant Nineteenth- and early 20th-century term for staff working with patients in asylums and workhouses.

autism A lifelong developmental condition that influences how a person communicates with and relates to other people, and how they make sense of the world around them.

autistic spectrum disorder Because autism can manifest itself in many different ways and has many different forms, the full range of conditions are known by some as a spectrum.

bagatelle A game in which small balls are propelled into numbered holes on a board, with pins as obstructions. The forerunner of pinball.

Bede houses Another term for almshouses.

Bedlam/Bethlem Popular names used by the public for the Royal Bethlehem Hospital in London, the first English institution for people with mental illness.

beggar A destitute person seeking money or help from members of the public.

Black Death A bubonic plague pandemic which ravished Europe, Asia and North Africa from 1346 to 1353, killing many millions of people. Possibly half of the population of England died as a result.

Bloody Code The name given retrospectively to the English justice system of the 18th century, which carried the harshest penalties, including death and transportation, for a very wide range of offences, many of which would be seen as only minor misdemeanours today.

blynde Early English word for blind.

Board of Control (for lunacy and mental deficiency) Government body established under the Mental Deficiency Act 1913 to replace the Lunacy Commission and to oversee the treatment of mentally ill people and people with learning disabilities.

Braidwoodian system A form of sign language (also known as the combined system) introduced by Thomas Braidwood, who set up the first academy for the deaf and dumb in London in 1783. The forerunner of British Sign Language.

Bridewell Originally a type of hospital, first established in the 16th century, for the improvement of the 'idle poor'. Eventually became 'houses of correction' for beggars and petty criminals.

British Sign Language (BSL) The sign language used in the United Kingdom and the preferred language of many deaf people in the UK.

care in the community A system of care and support for disabled people and people with mental illness based on the belief that people should live in their communities rather than in separate institutions. The Care in the Community Green Paper of 1981 signalled the end of the asylum era.

charitable asylum An asylum established as an independent charity through the voluntary efforts of members of the public. Popular at the end of the 18th and beginning of the 19th centuries before state asylums became the norm.

chronic lunatic Nineteenth-century term for a person with mental illness who is perceived as unlikely to recover from their illness.

City of London The original walled city (known today as the Square Mile), around which the greater conurbation of London later grew. Had its own system of government and was politically influential, particularly from the medieval period to the 18th century.

colony A type of asylum institution established by the 1913 Mental Deficiency Act where both adults and children with learning disabilities lived in a 'village' arrangement of a number of 'villas' each housing up to 60 people.

combined system A form of sign language (also known as the Braidwoodian system) introduced by Thomas Braidwood, who set up the first academy for the deaf and dumb in London in 1783. The forerunner of British Sign Language.

conglomerate asylum A form of asylum consisting of miscellaneous structures, without any real unity of style and often composed of buildings of widely varying ages.

corridor asylum A form of asylum consisting of a series of connecting corridors with wards and other rooms opening off them.

cosmos Another word for the universe, which carries a view of the universe as a complex, orderly and regulated system (*see* microcosm).

county lunatic asylums Asylums built by counties across England to house 'pauper lunatics and idiots', meaning mentally ill and learning-disabled people unable to meet the costs of their own care. From 1845 it was compulsory for counties to build such asylums, and many built more than one.

Court of Wards A court established in the Tudor period which allocated responsibility for the affairs of 'lunatics' and 'natural fools'.

cripple/creple A term used to describe physically disabled people until the second half of the 20th century (creple is its early English form, used in the medieval period). Now used pejoratively or abusively.

crooked/crookedness An early English term to describe people seen as misshapen in their bodily form.

curds and whey A sweet dish made from curdled milk products, sold as street food by vendors and hawkers in early modern England.

daily living skills The skills seen as necessary to be able to live an independent life, such as cooking, eating, budgeting, shopping and travelling. Restoration of daily living skills is often the focus of rehabilitation programmes.

deaf and dumb Often used to refer to deaf people who also had vocal communication problems, from the medieval to the modern period, but now no longer seen as appropriate terminology (*see also* dumbe).

deaff Early English word for deaf.

defective Term used in the early 20th century to describe a person who would be described today as having a learning disability.

deficient *See* mental deficiency.

degeneration/degenerate A theory propounded by eugenicists in the late 19th and 20th centuries. They believed that 'breeding' by disabled people, mentally ill people or people seen as 'feckless' or 'idle', particularly those from the poorer classes, would cause general racial deterioration in a society.

disabled access The design features or adaptations of a building such as ramps, doors, toilets etc which mean that disabled people can enter and make use of it.

dissolution The period largely between 1533 and 1545 when England under Henry VIII broke with the Church in Rome and 'dissolved' or plundered and shut down many religious buildings, including those which cared for the sick and the disabled.

dumbe Early English word for a person unable to speak (modern equivalent is *dumb*). From the medieval period till the 18th century it could signify that a person was deaf as well as unable to speak.

early modern Usually refers to the 16th, 17th and 18th centuries, the bridge between the medieval period and the 'modern' period.

empowerment The idea that disabled people should be in a position to have power and control over their own lives.

Enlightenment A period from the end of the 17th century through to the end of the 18th, when Western thinkers promoted the idea of reason and scientific knowledge as the basis of human happiness and social stability, and introduced new ideas of human freedom, progress, and toleration.

epilepsy A neurological disorder which can cause loss of consciousness or convulsions. Originally known as 'falling sickness'.

eugenics A movement prevalent in the later half of the 19th century and first half of the 20th century. Based on the writings of Francis Galton, eugenicists believed in the sterilisation or even euthanasia of disabled people and others such as the mentally ill or 'morally degenerate' to prevent what they described as racial deterioration. They believed that degeneration was due to genetic inheritance.

falling sickness Early English term for epilepsy.

feeble-minded A term used in the late 19th and early 20th centuries for people who would be described as having moderate or mild learning disabilities today or, as it was also known at the time, 'high-grade mental deficiency'. Offensive in modern parlance.

fool/foolish Early English word usually used to denote a person we would recognise as having a learning disability today. Could sometimes be used to denote a mentally ill person also. Also described people in the role of jester, but distinction was made between 'artificial fools', people pretending to be foolish, and 'natural fools', people born 'foolish'. Offensive in modern parlance.

furious Used in the 18th and 19th centuries to describe mentally ill people who are in a state of agitation or who are perceived to be potentially violent.

Georgian Used to describe the period from 1714 to 1830 in Britain when Britain was ruled by the Hanoverian dynasty. All four kings in the period were named George.

Great Exhibition The first World Fair, held in Hyde Park in London in 1851, to exhibit culture and industry from around the world. Organised by, among others, Prince Albert, the husband of Queen Victoria.

Guy's A hospital in London founded by the philanthropist Thomas Guy, initially a hospital for 'incurables'.

go-cart (or kart) An 18th-century slang expression to describe a disabled beggar who used a wooden box on wheels to move around.

Gordon riots Serious riots which took place in London in June 1780 to protest at the relaxation of anti-Catholic laws which had taken place two years earlier. Mainly targeted Catholic businesses and properties.

Hansen's disease The modern medical term for leprosy.

Harlequin Comic fool character identifiable by a particular form of chequered costume.

harlot Early English word for a prostitute.

humanist A practitioner of humanism, a movement which emerged from the so-called Italian Renaissance of the 15th and 16th centuries, which revived classical learning to place the human being at the centre of their own destiny, and human values at the centre of people's lives. While not rejecting religion, it challenged existing Christian thinking and brought about significant social change.

idiocy/idiot When classification systems were introduced in the 19th century, idiot was used to denote the lowest rank of intelligence and functional ability, similar to what we would define as a profound learning disability today. In earlier English used to describe 'dull-witted' people who could be seen as broadly equivalent to what we would define as learning disabled, but could be used in a wider sense to describe the labouring classes and the peasantry. Today used pejoratively or abusively.

imbecile When classification systems were introduced in the 19th century, imbecile was used to denote the medium rank of intelligence and functional ability among people with learning disabilities, between 'idiot' and 'moron'. Similar to what might be defined as a severe learning disability today. In the 19th century could also be used to describe a person with mental illness. Today used pejoratively or abusively.

impotent In its early English sense referred to people considered unable to look after themselves for reasons of age, infirmity or disability. The 'impotent poor' were distinguished from the 'able-bodied' or 'vagabond' poor in Poor Law legislation.

inaccessible Describes a building or area that a disabled person is unable to get into or use because its design prevents them from doing so.

incurable Term used to describe mentally ill or learning-disabled people whose condition was perceived to be permanent and who were therefore unable to 'recover'.

indigent blind Used in the 18th century to describe needy or poor blind people. The first charitable blind schools were for the 'indigent blind'.

industrial rehabilitation Rehabilitation for people injured or disabled in industrial accidents.

infirmary hall The section of medieval hospitals where the sick were treated, in sight of the chapel.

innocent Early English word for a 'natural fool', broadly a person we would recognise as having a learning disability today.

insane General term, still in use but not as widely as in the past, to denote mental illness. Tends to be associated with criminal or highly irrational behaviour, or often used pejoratively or abusively in current public usage.

institution A building used specifically for the separate care or treatment of specific groups of people, separated from mainstream society, and, usually, highly regulated in its operations.

keeper In the 16th and 17th centuries referred to any male carer, and did not imply any qualification.

lame/lameness Early English term meaning restricted use of one or more limbs. Applied to restricted use of arms as well as legs.

lazar house Medieval term for a specialist institution housing lepers (now known as people with Hansen's disease) derived from the name of the biblical character Lazarus.

learning disability The current terminology in use to describe the condition previously known as mental handicap, mental deficiency and many other terms. Usually denotes some form of intellectual impairment and problems in social functioning or coping with everyday basic skills.

leper house/hospital Medieval institution to house and care for people with leprosy (known today as Hansen's disease).

lepre/lepra Medieval terms for leper and leprosy respectively.

leprosy/leper Respectively, terms for the disease known today as Hansen's disease and those who have the disease. Highly prevalent disabling condition in England and the rest of Europe in the medieval period.

lesions General term for abnormalities in tissues of an organism, often caused by injury or disease. A common consequence of leprosy.

Lunacy Commission A public body established by the Lunacy Act of 1845 to oversee the welfare of people with mental illness ('lunatics') and people with learning disabilities ('idiots'). One of their roles was to monitor and inspect asylums.

lunatic/lunatick Early term broadly equivalent to the term 'mentally ill' used today. Current usage is pejorative or abusive.

mad doctor Eighteenth-century term to describe the proprietor or superintendent of a 'madhouse'. Mad doctors were not necessarily medically qualified.

madhouse A type of institution which began at the end of the 17th century and was particularly prevalent in the 18th century. Private houses which cared for and treated people with mental illness. Mostly treated private patients with independent means, but some also provided for 'pauper' patients paid for by parishes.

mainstream education Generally available public education ostensibly aimed at all children, but which often excludes disabled children.

Maison Dieu Literally 'Godly house', an alternative term for an almshouse.

mariners Early English word for sailors.

mental deficiency A term used mainly in the first part of the 20th century and broadly having the same meaning as the current term 'learning disability'.

mental handicap A term used mainly in the second half of the 20th century and broadly having the same meaning as the current term 'learning disability'.

mental health The state of a person's mental wellbeing.

mental illness The generally accepted current terminology for people who are seen as having some sort of health condition involving changes in emotion, thinking or behaviour (or a combination of these). In the past, certain types of mental illness were often referred to as lunacy or madness.

Metropolitan Asylums Board Established in 1867 under the Metropolitan Poor Act to care for London's 'sick poor'. Established about 40 institutions, including fever hospitals and 3 large purpose-built institutions for 'harmless and incurable lunatics' known as 'idiot asylums'. Duties passed to London County Council in 1930.

microcosm Something which captures in miniature the characteristics of something much larger. Embedded in the medieval and early modern view that there was a structural similarity between the human body and the wider cosmos (*see* cosmos).

mobility A person's ability to move around. Mobility aids and adaptations, such as wheelchairs, crutches and grab rails, and mobility vehicles such as scooters and adapted cars, are designed to assist people with restricted mobility.

Mongol/Mongolism/Mongolian imbecility The terms used by John Langdon Down, the 19th-century physician, to describe people known today as having Down syndrome. Derived from a belief (since discredited) that their facial features suggested some sort of ancient racial link to Mongolian people. Now unacceptable and abusive terms.

moral deficiency/morally deficient A category of people defined in the early 20th century broadly similar to moral imbecility, whose perceived 'deficiencies' were seen as linked to genetic inheritance.

moral imbecility/moral imbecile A category influenced by the ideas of eugenics in the early 20th century and contained in the 1913 Mental Deficiency Act. It labelled as a type of 'feeble-mindedness' those people who were believed not to be able to distinguish right from wrong. Drawn exclusively from the poorer classes, this category might include people who would be seen today as having mild learning disabilities. However, it could also include people such as prostitutes, mothers of illegitimate children and criminals.

moral management/treatment A method of treatment for people living in madhouses or lunatic asylums which rejected physical restraint and harsh treatment in favour of gentle discipline, order and therapeutic intervention. Pioneered by the Quaker York Retreat and taken up in some public asylums, in particular by John Connolly at Hanwell Asylum in the 19th century.

moron When classification systems were introduced in the 19th century, moron was used, particularly in the United States, to denote the higher rank of intelligence and functional ability among people with learning disabilities, above 'idiot' and 'imbecile'. Similar to what is defined as a moderate learning disability today. Today used pejoratively or abusively.

mystic A person who claims communion with God and prone to revelatory visions.

natural Shortened term for a natural fool.

natural fool Used from the medieval period until its usage died out in the 18th century to describe a person born with a lifelong mental impairment. Used to make a distinction from 'lunatics', seen as people suffering a temporary impairment due to mental illness. Also distinguished from 'artificial fool', someone pretending to be a fool, such as a court jester.

Norman A population from the Normandy region of France who conquered England in 1066, led by William the Conquerer, and brought about significant changes in law, finance, politics, architecture, religious practice, language and culture.

nurse In the 16th and 17th centuries referred to any paid carer, and did not imply any sort of qualification or training.

onanism Masturbation.

open-air school A type of school introduced to England from Germany in the early 20th century, where pupils spent much of their time learning outdoors. It was believed that fresh air would be beneficial to 'delicate' and disabled children.

ophthalmia An infection causing inflammation of the eye, previously a major cause of blindness but now treatable.

Origin of Species 1859 book by the naturalist Charles Darwin which introduced his theory of evolution, that all animal and human life has evolved from a common origin through a process of natural selection and adaptation over many millions of years. It undermined and represented a significant challenge to previous religious theories of human origin.

Paralympics Major international multisport event in which athletes with physical disabilities compete. Originated in England in 1948 as an event for disabled war veterans, and now a major world sporting event.

paralytic Early English word for paralysed.

parish A district for the purposes of local government, of particular importance from the medieval period through to the 19th century. Replaced by local authority boundaries. Originally defined by the area served by a church and priest.

pauper Early word for a person who does not have the means to support themselves, or who is in receipt of poor relief.

pavilion asylum A form of asylum characterised by parallel rows of uniform blocks each housing between 150 and 200 patients. The parallel rows separated male and female patients.

physiotherapy A healthcare profession which seeks to repair or improve impairments and disabilities through the promotion of mobility, functional ability and quality of life by physical intervention.

polio Poliomyelitis, an infectious viral disease affecting the central nervous system which can cause temporary or permanent paralysis. First identified in the 19th century, there were major epidemics across Europe throughout the 20th century. A common childhood disease and cause of disability in England until its eradication through a vaccination programme which began in the 1960s.

Poor Law Legislation designed to define English society's obligations and duties to the destitute, aged, sick or disabled people who were judged unable to look after themselves. Also contained punitive measures aimed at non-disabled poor people deemed 'idle' or unwilling to work. Began with a 1531 law under Henry VIII and culminated in the Poor Law Amendment Act of 1834.

poor relief From the 16th century, the use of parish or state funds to support destitute, sick, aged or disabled people, as stipulated by the Poor Law. Could be given as cash (outdoor relief) to allow people to achieve a level of subsistence needed for survival, or in kind (indoor relief), such as a place in a workhouse. After the 1834 Poor Law Amendment Act, indoor relief was favoured over outdoor relief.

Prerogativa Regis A 13th-century government document meaning 'prerogative of the king', which allowed kings to take possession of the lands and assets of people deemed to be 'idiots' or 'lunatics'.

Prince Albert (1819–61) The husband of Queen Victoria, known as the Prince Consort.

prior A prior (from the Latin for 'first') was a high-ranking person in the abbeys and monasteries of religious orders.

prosthetics The use of artificial replacements for missing body parts, particularly limbs.

psychiatrist A specially qualified doctor whose speciality is the study and treatment of mental illness.

psychologist A specialist who studies the human mind and its functions, particularly those affecting human behaviour in given contexts.

public assistance institution The term used in the 20th century to describe a workhouse.

purges The practice popular in early medicine, particularly in the 18th century, of removing blood or other fluids, eg vomit, from a patient. Derived from the idea that the health of a person depends on the balance of four 'humours', and that purging can restore balance when it has gone out of alignment.

purgatory In medieval belief a place of temporary suffering where people's earthly sins are cleansed before they ascend to heaven.

quack doctor A person pretending to have medical skills and promoting the sale of unproven or fraudulent medical remedies.

Quakers A religious movement originating in England in the 17th century, based on a belief in a direct relationship between individual believers and God. Quakers became prominent in social reform movements in the 18th century, including the establishment of humane asylums practising 'moral treatment'.

raving Early English word used to describe people experiencing episodes of mental illness where they appear to have no control of their emotions and to be talking nonsensically.

rehabilitation A process of medical and other interventions to enable people who have become disabled through accident or injury, or who have experienced mental illness, to recover skills and functions they have lost, to aid their recovery and reintegration into society.

relief *See* poor relief.

reserved occupations An idea introduced in legislation after the Second World War where certain jobs, such as lift attendants or car park attendants, were reserved solely for people with some sort of disability. Intended to boost employment of disabled people.

restraint The practice of using manacles, straitjackets or other physically coercive methods to control people seen as out of control, disruptive or dangerous.

retreat An early word to describe an isolated therapeutic environment, separate from the pressures of mainstream society, where people who have experienced mental illness can undergo healing and recovery (eg The York Retreat).

self-direction The idea that disabled people should be given funds with which to purchase and control their own support and care arrangements.

sheltered work Work for disabled people taking place in specialist work settings separate from mainstream workplaces.

shrine A holy or sacred place dedicated to a particular saint. In medieval England it was believed that many shrines were sites where miracle cures for different types of disability might take place, and therefore many disabled people were part of pilgrimages to shrines seeking cure.

sledge beggar An 18th-century expression to describe a disabled beggar who used a wooden sledge, pulled by a dog or another person, to move around.

social model The social model of disability argues that while physical, intellectual or social variations can cause individual limitations or impairments, it is society's failure to take account of these differences and include people that causes disability. The idea developed between the 1960s and 1980s in opposition to the 'medical model' of disability.

spastic The word originally used to describe a person with cerebral palsy, but now only used in a pejorative or abusive sense.

special education The provision of separate education in schools specifically established for children with disabilities (and other difficulties such as behaviour).

spinal paralysis Injury or damage to the spine causing the loss of the use of two limbs (paraplegic) or all four limbs (quadriplegic).

spital/spytall Early English word for a hospital.

sterilisation Surgical procedure to make men or women infertile. Advocated by the eugenics movement for people viewed as mentally and sometimes physically or morally degenerate or deficient.

sturdy Early English word meaning 'non-disabled' as in 'sturdy vagabond', meaning a beggar who has no disability or sickness preventing them from working.

Telethon The Telethons were three 27-hour-long charity fundraising events organised by the British television broadcaster ITV between 1988 and 1992. They were criticised by disability activists for representing disabled people as objects of pity and not involving them in events which were about them.

tickets porter A licensed street porter in London.

Tom o' Bedlam Sixteenth- and 17th-century expression to describe a mentally ill beggar.

trade guild Association of craftsmen in a particular trade, originating in the medieval period. The purpose of trade guilds was both to protect and regulate their own trade and to care for their own members, eg through the provision of almshouses.

tubercular Having tuberculosis, an infectious disease of the lungs.

ulcerations Open sores on the body, one of the symptoms of leprosy in the medieval period.

universal design Architectural approach which seeks to ensure that buildings are fully accessible in all parts to anyone with any sort of disability.

vagabond Early English word for a beggar, tending to denote those who were perceived as 'idle', dangerous or criminal, as opposed to impotent beggars who were incapacitated in some way and not seen as dangerous.

villa Used to describe the separate ward buildings housing up to 60 people in pavilion design asylums, particularly mental deficiency colonies.

ward of court *See* Court of Wards

water tower The high towers often at the centre of 19th-century asylums, and visible from a distance, which supplied water to asylum staff and patients. They became an iconic symbol of the separateness of the asylum.

wheelchair polo A form of the game of polo, which is usually played by riders on horses striking a ball with long mallets. Played instead in wheelchairs using shortened mallets. First played at Stoke Mandeville hospital.

workhouse An institution to house and put to work the destitute poor. Many destitute sick, aged and disabled people also lived in them. After the 1834 Poor Law Amendment Act, workhouses were deliberately designed as punitive and uncomfortable institutions to discourage people from 'idleness'.

Recommended reading

General history of disability

Two recent collections offer global perspectives over the span of history:

Bolt, D, and McRuer, R (eds) 2020 *A Cultural History of Disability* (6 volumes).
     London: Bloomsbury

Hanes, R, Brown, I, and Hansen, N E (eds) 2020 *The Routledge History of Disability*.
     London: Routledge

Theory

Disability theory is a dense and growing field. These books include some of the most important 'founding texts', while others offer the most accessible general introduction to the issues.

Goffman, E 1961 *Asylums: Essays on the Social Situation of Mental Patients and Other
     Inmates*. London: Penguin

Mitchell, D T, and Snyder, S L 2000 *Narrative Prosthesis: Disability and the
     Dependencies of Discourse*. Ann Arbor: University of Michigan Press

Oliver, M 1990 *The Politics of Disablement*. Basingstoke: Macmillan Press

Oliver, M, and Barnes, C 1998 *Disabled People and Social Policy: From Exclusion to
     Inclusion*. London: Longman

Shakespeare, T 2006 *Disability Rights and Wrongs*. Abingdon: Routledge

Shakespeare, T 2014 *Disability Rights and Wrongs Revisited*. Abingdon: Routledge

Wolfensberger, W 1975 *The Origin and Nature of our Institutionalized Models*. New
     York: Human Policy Press

Medieval period

There is a growing body of fine work on this period, and these are four of the finest.

Metzler, I 2006 *Disability in Medieval Europe: Thinking about Physical Impairment
     during the High Middle Ages*. Abingdon: Routledge

Metzler, I 2013 *A Social History of Disability in the Middle Ages: Cultural Considerations
     of Physical Impairment*. Abingdon: Routledge

Metzler, I 2016 *Fools and Idiots? Intellectual Disability in the Middle Ages*. Manchester:
     Manchester University Press

Rawcliffe, C 2006 *Leprosy in Medieval England*. Woodbridge: Boydell

16th and 17th centuries

The most unexplored of all the periods but MacDonald's work on mental illness in the 17th century is a classic, and Vincent-Connolly's recent work offers an interesting introduction.

MacDonald, M 1981 *Mystical Bedlam: Madness, Anxiety and Healing in 17th-Century England*. Cambridge: Cambridge University Press

Vincent-Connolly, P 2021 *Disability and the Tudors: All the King's Fools*. Barnsley: Pen and Sword

18th century

An excellent introduction to the range of disabilities and how they were understood and perceived in this period.

Turner, D 2012 *Disability in 18th-Century England: Imagining Physical Impairment*. London: Routledge

19th century

Kevles offers an introduction to the ideas and currents of thought which brought about eugenics, and Scull's is one of the best known and most comprehensive accounts of the asylum period.

Kevles, D 1995 *In the Name of Eugenics: Genetics and the Use of Human Heredity*. Cambridge, MA: Harvard University Press

Scull, A 1993 *The Most Solitary of Afflictions: Madness and Society in Britain, 1700–1900*. New Haven: Yale University Press

20th century

There is obviously a very wide range of texts on more recent history, but a good entry point is Julie Anderson's work on the impact of war. To get an understanding of social attitudes and everyday life experiences, Humphries and Gordon's collection of interviews with disabled people is unforgettable.

Anderson, J 2011 *War, Disability and Rehabilitation in Britain: 'Soul of a Nation'*. Manchester: Manchester University Press

Humphries, S, and Gordon, P 1992 *Out of Sight: The Experience of Disability 1900–1950*. Plymouth: Northcote House

Web resources

Accentuate, A history of place – eight places, 800 years in the lives of deaf and disabled people. https://historyof.place/

Historic England, Disability in Time and Place – A History of Disability from 1050 to the current day. https://historicengland.org.uk/research/inclusive-heritage/disability-history/

UK Disability History Month. https://ukdhm.org/

Index

Page numbers in **bold** refer to figures.